Hideomi Watanabe · Misako Koizumi (eds.)

Advanced Initiatives in Interprofessional Education in Japan

Japan Interprofessional Working and Education Network

Hideomi Watanabe · Misako Koizumi (eds.)

Advanced Initiatives in Interprofessional Education in Japan

Japan Interprofessional Working and Education Network

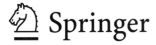

Editors
Hideomi Watanabe, M.D., Ph.D.
Department of Physical Therapy, School of Health Sciences
Gunma University
3-39-15 Showa, Maebashi 371-8511, Japan

Misako Koizumi, Ph.D.
Department of Nursing, School of Health Sciences
Gunma University
3-39-15 Showa, Maebashi 371-8511, Japan

ISBN: 978-4-431-98075-9   e-ISBN: 978-4-431-98076-6
DOI 10.1007/978-4-431-98076-6
Springer Tokyo Berlin Heidelberg New York

Library of Congress Control Number: 2009939423

© Springer 2010
This work is subject to copyright. All rights are reserved, whether the whole or part of the material is concerned, specifically the rights of translation, reprinting, reuse of illustrations, recitation, broadcasting, reproduction on microfilms or in other ways, and storage in data banks.
The use of registered names, trademarks, etc. in this publication does not imply, even in the absence of a specific statement, that such names are exempt from the relevant protective laws and regulations and therefore free for general use.
Product liability: The publisher can give no guarantee for information about drug dosage and application thereof contained in this book. In every individual case the respective user must check its accuracy by consulting other pharmaceutical literature.

Printed on acid-free paper

Springer is a part of Springer Science+Business Media (www.springer.com)

Preface

Deterioration in the quality of health professionals is a big concern in Japan. The deterioration is caused by the fact that in order to respond to a serious shortage, a large number of health workers have been produced rapidly without any effective quality assurance. As a means to improve the quality in health professions, there has been an upsurge of interest in interprofessional education (IPE) in academic institutions around the world. Much has been published on the subject in the last decade, mainly from the United Kingdom and other parts of Europe, the United States, Canada, and Australia. Japan, on the other hand, has published relatively little about IPE, in spite of the recognition of its significance by many health-care professionals and medical training institutions. Several Japanese institutions have recently developed and systemically implemented extensive IPE programs, however. The initiatives of these institutions have been approved as Good Practices by the Japanese government, and, as a result, financial support for their IPE programs has been obtained. The Japan Interprofessional Working and Education Network (JIPWEN) was established in June 2008 comprising ten universities.

JIPWEN aims to discuss critical IPE issues together and to present broadly applicable plural models so that institutions interested in the IPE programs can adapt those models to their own academic and social settings. Nowadays, more and more institutions are planning to start IPE activities. JIPWEN advocates and strengthens those activities, because IPE plays an important role in optimizing interprofessional work. JIPWEN does not aim to establish an association, which organizes meetings for open discussion with all educators or preceptors who are interested in IPE, but instead aims to connect them to government health policy planning and international networks. Most JIPWEN activities are planned and implemented in consultation and through cooperation with the World Health Organization (WHO) [http://jipwen.dept.showa.gunma-u.ac.jp]. JIPWEN is also a member of the Global Health Workforce Alliance (GHWA) [http://www.who.int/workforcealliance/en/].

This book consists of chapters from ten member-universities belonging to JIPWEN. Their programs vary in content, as do their individual backgrounds, goals, methods, modules, student compositions, facilitation systems, and timing of their respective university curricula. Programs of each institution are summarized in Annex 1. Interestingly, the backgrounds commonly depicted in most universities correspond well to the topics described in The World Health Report 2008 issued from WHO. Objectives or goals of the institutions' IPE programs include promotion of community health care, communication skills, and comprehensive health services. The experience of each institution is relatively brief, from 2 to 12 years, except for the Tokyo Jikeikai Medical University, which started its IPE program in 1989. All universities perform assessments of their IPE activities using their original evaluation systems, and most have shown significant results statistically. The purpose of this book is to describe, in detail, the diverse IPE programs implemented at the JIPWEN member institutions, and to provide plural models for the increasing number of institutions aiming to develop their own IPE programs.

In the way of acknowledgments, we are deeply grateful first of all to the Department of Human Resources for Health of the WHO for its generous cooperation in interprofessional education. We especially thank Mr. Hugo Mercer, former coordinator, and Dr. Alexandre Goubarev, scientist, of the Health Workforce Education and Production Team (HEP) for their advice and support in establishing a collaborative tie between WHO and JIPWEN.

We greatly value the extensive support of Gunma University academically, socially, and financially. We sincerely acknowledge Professor Kuniaki Takada, President of Gunma University; Professor Hiroo Hoshino, Dean of the Faculty of Medicine; and Professor Hirokazu Murakami, former Dean of the School of Health Sciences for their continuous and kind support. We are also indebted to Professor Seiji Ozawa, former Vice President of Gunma University, and Professor Osamu Ishikawa, Director of Gunma University Hospital, for their critical review and kind suggestions. We owe great thanks to the members of the Educational Committee of the School of Medicine of Gunma University, especially to Professor Jun-ichi Tamura, Chief of the Committee, and to Professor Noriyuki Koibuchi, Vice Chief of the Committee, for their kind and intense collaboration.

We are grateful for the valuable support received from the staff of the School of Health Sciences in the Educational Affairs Office, Showa Campus Administration Division, Gunma University, for their support in the planning of this book. In particular, we deeply thank Mr. Mutsuhito Yomoda, Mr. Shoji Ishimori, Mr. Kazuo Takahira, Ms. Mika Sato, and Ms. Kyoko Tsuda for their kind assistance in writing and editing.

Finally, we thank staff of Springer Japan, for her editorial assistance in publishing this book.

Hideomi Watanabe and Misako Koizumi, Editors
IEP Committee, Gunma University School of Health Sciences
Maebashi, Japan
November 2009

Contents

Preface V
Contributors IX

Encouraging Appreciation of Community Health Care by Consistent Medical Undergraduate Education
Community Health Care Training Beyond the University Hospital for Mutual Understanding Between Medical Students and the Community 1
H. Sohma, I. Sawada, M. Konno, H. Akashi, T.J. Sato, T. Maruyama, N. Tohse, and K. Imai

Interprofessional Education at Niigata University of Health and Welfare Implementation of an Integrated General Seminar and Future Prospects 13
R. Oshiki, A. Magara, E. Hoshino, Y. Nishihara, S. Masegi, E. Watanabe, M. Kaibuchi, Y. Nagai, and H.E. Takahashi

Interprofessional Education Program of the University of Tsukuba: A Program to Develop Interprofessional Competence 23
T. Maeno, A. Takayashiki, T. Maeno, T. Anme, A. Hara, Y. Saeki, O. Urayama, and F. Otsuka

Community-Based Interprofessional Education at Saitama Prefectural University 39
M. Otsuka, M. Shimazaki, K. Kayaba, T. Sakada, K. Hara, M. Asahi, T. Arai, I. Murohashi, K. Yokoyama, N. Hasegawa, M. Kawamata, R. Suzuki, C. Fujii, N. Kunisawa, M. Kanemune, N. Shimasue, H. Shinmura, K. Nishihara, K. Inoue, K. Ogawa, and R. Tano

Jikei University School of Medicine: An Interprofessional Medical Education Program 49
O. Fukushima

**Interprofessional Education at the Keio University
Faculty of Pharmacy** 57
*Y. Ehara, Y. Abe, K. Fujimoto, N. Fukushima, S. Iijima, S. Ishikawa,
K. Kishimoto, M. Mochizuki, K. Takahashi, E. Yokota, and S. Kobayashi*

**Support Program for Contemporary Educational Needs: "Contemporary
Good Practice" Project at Chiba University
Educational Program for Training Autonomous Health
Care Professionals: Human Resource Training Emphasizing
Interprofessional Collaboration** 65
*M. Miyazaki, I. Sakai, T. Majima, I. Ishii, Y. Sekine, M. Tanabe,
M. Asahina, H. Noguchi, N. Ide, and K. Iida (Chiba University
Inohana IPE Working Group)*

**Interprofessional Team-Based Medical Education Program at Kitasato
University: Collaboration Among 14 Health-Related Professions** 75
*K. Mizumoto, M. Okamoto, K. Ishii, M. Noshiro, Y. Kuroda, M. Shirataka,
M. Taga, K. Iguchi, H. Ikemoto, and T. Shiba*

Becoming Interprofessional at Kobe University 95
*Y. Tamura, Y. Ishikawa, P. Bontje, T. Shirakawa, H. Andou, I. Miyawaki,
K. Watanabe, Y. Miura, R. Ono, K. Hirata, M. Hirai, and K. Seki*

**Interprofessional Education Initiatives at Gunma University: Simulated
Interprofessional Training for Students of Various Health Science
Professions** 113
*H. Ogawara, T. Hayashi, Y. Asakawa, K. Iwasaki, T. Matsuda, Y. Abe,
F. Tozato, T. Makino, H. Shinozaki, M. Koizumi, T. Yasukawa, and
H. Watanabe*

Annex 130
Subject Index 137

Contributors

Abe, Yoshihiro
Faculty of Pharmacy, Keio University, Tokyo, Japan

Abe, Yumiko
Department of Laboratory Science, School of Health Sciences, Gunma University, Maebashi, Japan

Akashi, Hirofumi
Sapporo Medical University Scholarly Communication Center, Sapporo, Japan

Andou, Hiroshi
Kobe University Graduate School of Health Sciences, Kobe, Japan

Anme, Tokie
School of Nursing, School of Medicine and Medical Sciences, University of Tsukuba, Tsukuba, Japan

Arai, Toshitami
Department of Social Work, Saitama Prefectural University School of Health and Social Services, Koshigaya, Japan

Asahi, Masaya
Department of Social Work, Saitama Prefectural University School of Health and Social Services, Koshigaya, Japan

Asahina, Mayumi
School of Medicine, Graduate School of Medicine, Chiba University, Chiba, Japan

Asakawa, Yasuyoshi
Department of Physical Therapy, School of Health Sciences, Gunma University, Maebashi, Japan

Bontje, Peter
KIPEC (Kobe University Interprofessional Education for Collaborative Working Center), Kobe, Japan

Ehara, Yoshihiro
Faculty of Pharmacy, Keio University, Tokyo, Japan

Fujii, Chiyo
Department of Social Work, Saitama Prefectural University School of Health and Social Services, Koshigaya, Japan

Fujimoto, Kazuko
Faculty of Pharmacy, Keio University, Tokyo, Japan

Fukushima, Noriko
Faculty of Pharmacy, Keio University, Tokyo, Japan

Fukushima, Osamu
Center for Medical Education, Jikei University School of Medicine, Tokyo, Japan

Hara, Akira
School of Medicine, School of Medicine and Medical Sciences, University of Tsukuba, Tsukuba, Japan

Hara, Kazuhiko
Department of Physical Therapy, Saitama Prefectural University School of Health and Social Services, Koshigaya, Japan

Hasegawa, Naomi
Department of Nursing, Saitama Prefectural University School of Health and Social Services, Koshigaya, Japan

Hayashi, Tomoko
Department of Nursing, School of Health Sciences, Gunma University, Maebashi, Japan

Hirai, Midori
Department of Pharmacology, Kobe University Hospital, Kobe, Japan

Hirata, Kenichi
Kobe University, Graduate School of Medicine, Kobe, Japan

Hoshino, Emiko
Department of Social Welfare, Faculty of Social Welfare, Niigata University of Health and Welfare, Niigata, Japan

Ide, Narumi
School of Nursing, Graduate School of Nursing, Chiba University, Chiba, Japan

Iguchi, Kaoru
Kitasato Nursing School, Kitamoto, Japan

Iida, Kieko
School of Nursing, Graduate School of Nursing, Chiba University, Chiba, Japan

Iijima, Shiro
Faculty of Pharmacy, Keio University, Tokyo, Japan

Contributors

Ikemoto, Hisashi
Education Center, Kitasato University, Sagamihara, Japan

Imai, Kohzoh
Sapporo Medical University, Sapporo, Japan

Inoue, Kazuhisa
Department of Physical Therapy, Saitama Prefectural University School of Health and Social Services, Koshigaya, Japan

Ishii, Itsuko
Faculty of Pharmaceutical Sciences, Graduate School of Pharmaceutical Sciences, Chiba University, Chiba, Japan

Ishii, Kunio
School of Pharmacy, Kitasato University, Tokyo, Japan

Ishikawa, Satoko
Faculty of Pharmacy, Keio University, Tokyo, Japan

Ishikawa, Yuichi
Kobe University Graduate School of Health Sciences, Kobe, Japan

Iwasaki, Kiyotaka
Department of Occupational Therapy, School of Health Sciences, Gunma University, Maebashi, Japan

Kaibuchi, Masato
Department of Occupational Therapy, Faculty of Medical Technology, Niigata University of Health and Welfare, Niigata, Japan

Kanemune, Miyuki
Department of Nursing, Saitama Prefectural University School of Health and Social Services, Koshigaya, Japan

Kawamata, Minoru
Department of Physical Therapy, Saitama Prefectural University School of Health and Social Services, Koshigaya, Japan

Kayaba, Kazunori
Department of Health Sciences, Saitama Prefectural University School of Health and Social Services, Koshigaya, Japan

Kishimoto, Keiko
Faculty of Pharmacy, Keio University, Tokyo, Japan

Kobayashi, Shizuko
Faculty of Pharmacy, Keio University, Tokyo, Japan

Koizumi, Misako
Department of Nursing, School of Health Sciences, Gunma University, Maebashi, Japan

Konno, Miki
Department of Nursing, Sapporo Medical University, School of Health Sciences, Sapporo, Japan

Kunisawa, Naoko
Department of Health Sciences, Saitama Prefectural University School of Health and Social Services, Koshigaya, Japan

Kuroda, Yuko
School of Nursing, Kitasato University, Sagamihara, Japan

Maeno, Takami
School of Medicine, School of Medicine and Medical Sciences, University of Tsukuba, Tsukuba, Japan

Maeno, Tetsuhiro
School of Medicine, School of Medicine and Medical Sciences, University of Tsukuba, Tsukuba, Japan

Magara, Akira
Department of Prosthetics & Orthotics and Assistive Technology, Faculty of Medical Technology, Niigata University of Health and Welfare, Niigata, Japan

Majima, Tomoko
School of Nursing, Graduate School of Nursing, Chiba University, Chiba, Japan

Makino, Takatoshi
Department of Nursing, School of Health Sciences, Gunma University, Maebashi, Japan

Maruyama, Tomoko
Sapporo Medical University, School of Health Sciences, Sapporo, Japan

Masegi, Seiya
Department of Health and Sports, Faculty of Health Sciences, Niigata University of Health and Welfare, Niigata, Japan

Matsuda, Tamiko
Department of Nursing, School of Health Sciences, Gunma University, Maebashi, Japan

Miura, Yasushi
Kobe University Graduate School of Health Sciences, Kobe, Japan

Miyawaki, Ikuko
Kobe University Graduate School of Health Sciences, Kobe, Japan

Miyazaki, Misako
School of Nursing, Graduate School of Nursing, Chiba University, Chiba, Japan

Mizumoto, Kiyohisa
Kitasato University, Tokyo, Japan

Mochizuki, Mayumi
Faculty of Pharmacy, Keio University, Tokyo, Japan

Murohashi, Ikuo
Department of Health Sciences, Saitama Prefectural University School of Health and Social Services, Koshigaya, Japan

Nagai, Yoichi
Department of Occupational Therapy, Faculty of Medical Technology, Niigata University of Health and Welfare, Niigata, Japan

Nishihara, Ken
Department of Physical Therapy, Saitama Prefectural University School of Health and Social Services, Koshigaya, Japan

Nishihara, Yasuyuki
Department of Health and Sports, Faculty of Health Sciences, Niigata University of Health and Welfare, Niigata, Japan

Noguchi, Hotaka
School of Medicine, Graduate School of Medicine, Chiba University, Chiba, Japan

Noshiro, Makoto
School of Allied Health Sciences, Kitasato University, Sagamihara, Japan

Ogawa, Kumi
Department of Social Work, Saitama Prefectural University School of Health and Social Services, Koshigaya, Japan

Ogawara, Hatsue
Department of Laboratory Science, School of Health Sciences, Gunma University, Maebashi, Japan

Okamoto, Makito
School of Medicine, Kitasato University, Sagamihara, Japan

Ono, Rei
Kobe University Graduate School of Health Sciences, Kobe, Japan

Oshiki, Rieko
Department of Physiotherapy, Faculty of Medical Technology, Niigata University of Health and Welfare, Niigata, Japan

Otsuka, Fujio
School of Medicine, School of Medicine and Medical Sciences, University of Tsukuba, Tsukuba, Japan

Otsuka, Mariko
Department of Nursing, Saitama Prefectural University School of Health and Social Services, Koshigaya, Japan

Saeki, Yuka
School of Nursing, School of Medicine and Medical Sciences, University of Tsukuba, Tsukuba, Japan

Sakada, Takanori
Department of Nursing, Saitama Prefectural University School of Health and Social Services, Koshigaya, Japan

Sakai, Ikuko
School of Nursing, Graduate School of Nursing, Chiba University, Chiba, Japan

Sato, Toshio J.
Department of Educational Development, Sapporo Medical University Center for Medical Education, Japan

Sawada, Izumi
Department of Nursing, Sapporo Medical University, School of Health Sciences, Sapporo, Japan

Seki, Keiko
Kobe University Graduate School of Health Sciences, Kobe, Japan

Sekine, Yuko
Faculty of Pharmaceutical Sciences, Graduate School of Pharmaceutical Sciences, Chiba University, Chiba, Japan

Shiba, Tadayoshi
Kitasato University, Tokyo, Japan

Shimasue, Noriko
Department of Social Work, Saitama Prefectural University School of Health and Social Services, Koshigaya, Japan

Shimazaki, Midori
Department of Social Work, Saitama Prefectural University School of Health and Social Services, Koshigaya, Japan

Shinmura, Hiromi
Department of Nursing, Saitama Prefectural University School of Health and Social Services, Koshigaya, Japan

Shinozaki, Hiromitsu
Department of Nursing, School of Health Sciences, Gunma University, Maebashi, Japan

Shirakawa, Taku
Kobe University Graduate School of Health Sciences, Kobe, Japan

Shirataka, Masuo
College of Liberal Arts and Sciences, Kitasato University, Sagamihara, Japan

Sohma, Hitoshi
Department of Educational Development, Sapporo Medical University Center for Medical Education, Sapporo, Japan

Suzuki, Reiko
Department of Nursing, Saitama Prefectural University School of Health and Social Services, Koshigaya, Japan

Taga, Masaki
Kitasato Junior College of Health and Hygienic Sciences, Niigata, Japan

Takahashi, Hideaki E.
Niigata University of Health and Welfare, Niigata, Japan

Takahashi, Kyoko
Faculty of Pharmacy, Keio University, Tokyo, Japan

Takayashiki, Ayumi
School of Medicine, School of Medicine and Medical Sciences, University of Tsukuba, Tsukuba, Japan

Tamura, Yumi
Kobe University Graduate School of Health Sciences, Kobe, Japan

Tanabe, Masahiro
School of Medicine, Graduate School of Medicine, Chiba University, Chiba, Japan

Tano, Rumi
Department of Health Sciences, Saitama Prefectural University School of Health and Social Services, Koshigaya, Japan

Tohse, Noritsugu
Sapporo Medical University School of Medicine, Sapporo, Japan

Tozato, Fusae
Department of Occupational Therapy, School of Health Sciences, Gunma University, Maebashi, Japan

Urayama, Osamu
School of Medical Sciences, School of Medicine and Medical Sciences, University of Tsukuba, Tsukuba, Japan

Watanabe, Eikichi
Department of Health and Nutrition, Faculty of Health Sciences, Niigata University of Health and Welfare, Niigata, Japan

Watanabe, Hideomi
Department of Physical Therapy, School of Health Sciences, Gunma University, Maebashi, Japan

Watanabe, Kaori
Kobe University Graduate School of Health Sciences, Kobe, Japan

Yasukawa, Takako
Department of Physical Therapy, School of Health Science, Gunma University, Maebashi, Japan; Department of Internal Medicine, Seirei Hamamatsu General Hospital, Hamamatsu, Japan

Yokota, Eriko
Faculty of Pharmacy, Keio University, Tokyo, Japan

Yokoyama, Keiko
Department of Nursing, Saitama Prefectural University School of Health and Social Services, Koshigaya, Japan

Encouraging Appreciation of Community Health Care by Consistent Medical Undergraduate Education

Community Health Care Training Beyond the University Hospital for Mutual Understanding Between Medical Students and the Community

Hitoshi Sohma[1], **Izumi Sawada**[2], **Miki Konno**[2], **Hirofumi Akashi**[3], **Toshio J. Sato**[1], **Tomoko Maruyama**[4], **Noritsugu Tohse**[5], and **Kohzoh Imai**[6]

Summary

Hokkaido Prefecture of Japan covers a vast geographical area. The uneven distribution of medical personnel in Hokkaido is accountable for the scarcity of medical services in certain areas. As a result, the anxiety of the population living in those underserved areas increases, thereby posing a serious social concern. The interprofessional education (IPE) program was proposed as a response to a concern about community health care. This program was meant to systematize various practical experience training programs and restructure them into one joint curriculum for community health care, in addition to expanding the residential community internship program. This enables the entire university to undertake consistent education on community health. The residential community and team-based training programs aim at producing professionals who will serve in the community. These programs encourage students to have an interest in community health as professionals

---

[1] Department of Educational Development, Sapporo Medical University Center for Medical Education, South-1, West-17, Chuo-ku, Sapporo 060-8556, Japan
Tel. +81-11-611-2111 (ext. 2370); Fax +81-11-611-2139
e-mail: sohma@sapmed.ac.jp
[2] Department of Nursing, Sapporo Medical University, School of Health Sciences, Sapporo, Japan
[3] Sapporo Medical University Scholarly Communication Center, Sapporo, Japan
[4] Sapporo Medical University, School of Health Sciences, Sapporo, Japan
[5] Sapporo Medical University School of Medicine, Sapporo, Japan
[6] Sapporo Medical University, Sapporo, Japan

Correspondence to: H. Sohma

through practice training during their initial school years. Furthermore, the residential joint curriculum (team-based residential community health care internship) provides students with an opportunity to interact not only with medical professionals but also patients and their families and health care staff. This leads to opening their eyes to disease prevention specifically and more widely to community issues. Through IPE, students are expected to: (1) strengthen their interest in community health care, which they have had even upon entry to the university; (2) deepen their understanding of the community, particularly community health care; (3) obtain an appreciation toward and a sense of empowerment within community health care; and (4) develop a sense of mission and deep commitment to community health care.

Key words Appreciation of community health care · Joint curriculum · Consistent education in community health care · Team-based medicine · Partnership

1 Profile of the University

Sapporo Medical University was founded as the Hokkaido prefectural medical college in 1950; thus, it has a history of about 60 years. The university's mottoes during its formative era were "a spirit of challenge in an open-minded interaction" and "pursuit of medical sciences and health care and contribution to community health care." To have the concepts behind these mottoes materialize, the university has based its fundamental principles on practical, highly specialized education to bring forth professionals who will serve the community. In 1993, a new School of Health Science, which includes the departments of nursing, physiotherapy, and occupational therapy, was added, thus making the college a medical university.

To date, the university has a number of achievements, including high recruitment and retention rates of its graduates in the prefecture. Both schools have been carrying out facility and clinical training with community health care as the primary focus. During the fiscal year (FY) 2004, its community-based training was awarded one of the Grant-in-Aid programs (called modern good practice, or modern GP) supported by the Ministry of Education, Culture, Sports, Science, and Technology of Japan; it has further strengthened our educational initiatives for community health care. For instance, the university recently initiated a residential team-based internship program that is specifically tailored for students who intend to work in the community. Under the program, all four departments (i.e., one from the School of Medicine and three from the School of Health Science) join into teams and go through training in these teams—a program called interprofessional education (IPE). In addition, the university has been carrying out a medical personnel training program, called medical personnel GP, aimed at skills improvement and a better preparation of doctors who will serve the community. Furthermore, in FY2005 we implemented an innovative educational program in support of intellectual property of medical researchers and community health care practitioners. By FY2006, we adopted another experimental educational program that cuts across high school and university curricula and aims at more efficient professional training.

2 Background and Goals of IPE

2.1 Background

Hokkaido Prefecture covers a vast geographical area. The uneven distribution of medical personnel in Hokkaido is responsible for the scarcity of medical services in certain areas. As a result, the anxiety of the population living in those underserved areas increases, posing a serious social concern. Although the number of medical doctors per 100 000 population for the overall prefecture is above the national average of 211.7, most of the doctors are concentrated in urban areas such as Sapporo and Asahikawa. In fact, many public hospitals in other parts of the prefecture suffer from a chronic shortage of medical doctors. At the moment, 37% of the hospitals in the prefecture have unfilled vacancies for medical doctors (Table 1).

This is also the case for nurses and co-medical staff. The Seven-to-One Basic Fee for Hospitalization Rule that was newly introduced under the medical fee revision in April 2006 further aggravated the maldistribution of hospital nurses between urban and rural areas (Table 1). Public health nurses are increasingly expected to serve complex and diverse needs of communities. To do so, they must be equipped with specialized skills that should be supported through proper career development. Ensuring the number and quality of public health nurses is an imperative that is expected to be achieved through tight coordination between the university and communities. Similarly, occupational therapists and physical therapists are concentrated in urban areas. Roughly half of them are in and around Sapporo, whereas about 40% of the towns and the villages in the prefecture have neither of the two, which poses a serious problem.

Today's health care is not just straightforward medical treatment. It involves various medical activities, including those in response to the following issues: (1) an increase in the number of people who require long-term nursing care owing to

Table 1. Numbers of doctors and nurses per 100 000 population

Region	No. of doctors/100 000 persons	No. of nurses and assistant nurses/100 000 persons
Kamikawa, central part	299.0	1348.1
Sapporo	265.9	1137.6
Soya	105.5	815.3
Nemuro	100.4	676.5
Whole country	211.7	897.6

Source: Hokkaido Government report in fiscal year 2005

the aging population; (2) an increase in the number of lifestyle-related illnesses; (3) the diversity and complexity of illnesses; (4) the increased demands of patients; and (5) the higher demands for better-quality medical care. To strengthen community health care, cooperation among various health professions is indispensable, and involvement of not only medical doctors but also a wide range of medical professionals is essential.

In our university, two initiatives have been undertaken by each of the two schools individually, aimed at preparing medical personnel who will serve the community. The first is a residential community internship program under which students are requested to stay at a remote community for a certain period of time. The second is a team-based training program under which students' capacity to cooperate with other professionals is expected to improve. By integrating the two programs, a joint curriculum of the two schools—a team-based residential community internship program—was initiated in FY2004. In addition to these programs, students go through a more specialized medical training program during the later academic years.

2.2 Goals

In addition to expanding the residential community internship program, IPE is meant to systematize various practical experience training programs and restructure them into one joint curriculum for community health care. This enables the entire university to undertake consistent education for community health. Through IPE, students are expected to: (1) strengthen their interest in community health care, which they must have had even upon entry to the university; (2) deepen their understanding of the community, particular community health care; (3) obtain an appreciation toward and a sense of empowerment within community health care; and (4) develop a sense of mission and deep commitment to community health care. Altogether, encouraging a fuller appreciation of the importance of community health care is the primary objective of IPE. To this end, IPE aims to nurture a mutual understanding with local residents (which is essential for good community health care practice) and the capacity to cooperate with various professionals (partnership capacity) (Fig. 1).

3 Details of IPE

3.1 Special Features of the Programs

3.1.1 Programs to Date and Framework for the Future

Traditionally, medical undergraduate students go through classwork on community health care in their initial years and then take the residential community health care

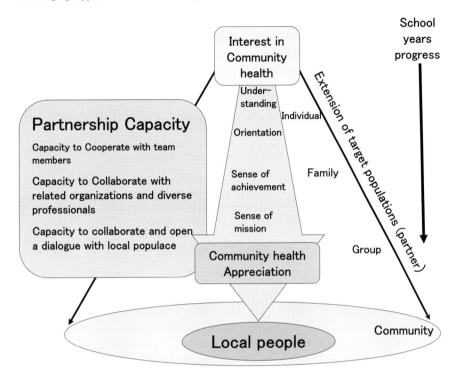

Fig. 1. Encouraging partnership and appreciation of community health. Many students enter a school with an interest in community health care. Certain steps are followed: (1) encouraging appreciation of community health care; understanding (understand) → orientation (let's do it) → feeling of achievement (we can) → sense of mission (we must). (2) Partnership capacity (interprofessional cooperation) with clear goals: equal relations among diverse professionals → optimizing expertise of professionals → collaboration and cooperation. Included are the individual (target populations) → family → community group → entire community of people

training (clinical training) in their fifth and sixth years. This is to ensure that consistency and continuity of education is maintained (Fig. 2). In the School of Health Sciences, the team-based practical training program has also been carried out systematically since the early years of its history. The introduction to medicine and the general theory of medicine at the Medical School and the general theory of health sciences at the School of Health Sciences are the primary threads of the education. To some extent, these courses help link various community health training programs in a coherent manner. The linkage among the various training programs, however, is not as strong as it should be. In fact, because each school carries out its respective practical training program separately (except for the team-based residential community internship program), continuity and consistency were missing from these programs, often ending up as isolated experiences for students. Hence, it has not been easy to create strong synergy and linkage between the practical training programs and classwork.

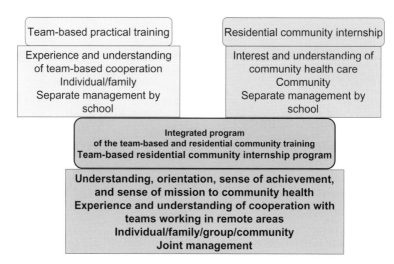

Fig. 2. Profiles of interprofessional education programs to date

The team-based residential community internship program is the first one jointly carried out by the two schools (IPE). It is a comprehensive undertaking intended to nurture students' orientation toward community health care and their capacity to cooperate as a team. The joint program, cutting across the boundaries of schools and departments, will bring about educational synergy, which is an obvious opportunity for a medical university such as ours to exploit through the necessary curriculum development.

The team-based residential community internship program uses the town of Betsukai-cho as its model community, as it is one of the towns in the prefecture suffering from the scarcity of medical services. Students from the medical department and from the three departments in the School of Health Sciences form a team; they stay in eastern Hokkaido (the Konsen district, which includes Betsukai-cho, Nakashibetsu-cho, and Kushiro-shi) and go through training. During the preparatory training period of 6 months prior to the main program, students take relevant classes taught not only by medical personnel but also by staff from the municipal administration. Using various materials, student groups also prepare themselves for the self-learning program and interactive seminars on health education. Thereafter, they start the program proper. Under the program, students improve their interpersonal communication skills through real-life and direct interactions with patients and target residents, leading to improved morale as medical professionals. Students also form groups and organize health education seminars for the prevention of diseases and the promotion of health, targeting local schoolchildren and the community's elderly (Fig. 3). This exercise helps students from different departments acquire fundamental professional ethics and attitudes to understand and respect other professionals. It also helps them appreciate the importance of community health care using the team-based approach, thereby increasing their motivation. The educational experience of sharing a significant amount of time with nonacademic

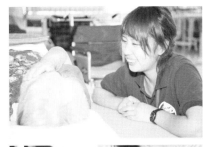
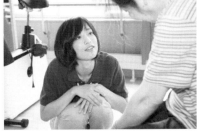
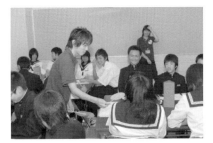
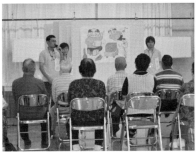

Joint team-based health care training by students from four department at medical and welfare facilities in Bekkai-cho and Kushiro City

Health education seminar in elementary school, junior high school, and clubs for the elderly (primary prevention education practice)

Fig. 3. Team-based residential community internship. Joint team-based health care training by students from four departments at medical and welfare facilities in Betsukai-cho and Kushiro

local community staff and residents helps students mature. This impact is increased with the students' living arrangements, whereby students from both schools/departments live and work together. The program induces communication opportunities with the academic staff, particularly those from other departments, thus exposing the students to diverse views.

As the next step, the joint team-based residential community internship program should be mainstreamed into the regular annual curriculum as a sustainable, consistent educational activity (development of a joint community health care seminar). By doing this, knowledge of community health care and related partnership arrangements can be systematized; the experiences of the team-based and residential community programs can be consolidated, leading to their eventual integration. In this way, it is possible to undertake educational activities in a sustainable way and systematically move the students toward a deeper appreciation of the importance of community health care (Fig. 4).

3.1.2 Educational Benefits

Although constraints on the educational curriculum exist, there have already been clinical training programs in local communities that provide practical opportunities

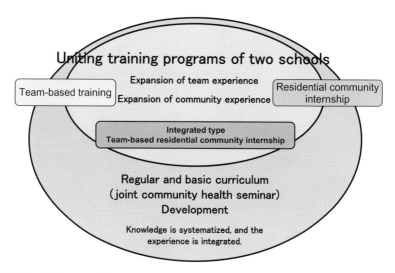

Fig. 4. Special features of the program

for students to learn off-site. These programs include not only traditional clinical training at medical facilities but also students' interactions and discussions with the staff of municipal health care and welfare administration and health centers; these experiences also include health education seminars targeting local residents (i.e., members of the local senior citizens' clubs, students of the local elementary and junior high schools) organized by students. Through such interactions and discussions, the students are able to grasp the issues that local communities face and come to understand local communities in a holistic manner (e.g., from medical, social, and economic perspectives). The joint program of the two schools features team-based clinical training through which students can learn the importance of a team-based approach that is essential for community health care, along with the respective roles of other professions. Therefore, further educational benefits can be expected by conducting more residential and joint team-based programs with the students.

The programs involve interactions with not only local medical facilities but also local administration offices, community circles, and local residents from all walks of life. This enables the community to better understand the university, its medical doctors, and other health care professionals. In fact, the cities, towns, and villages where the university is carrying out its residential internship programs have proven to be keener about health promotion and preventive medicine, more supportive of medical doctors, and by and large have stable, sound health services. In the future, more collaborative relations can be established with various local communities and the university by increasing the number of target communities of the program.

3.1.3 Tips for Motivating Students for Community Health Care

To ensure students' appreciation of community health care, it is important to train them systematically and consistently on community health right from their initial years of education (Table 2). In particular, conducting clinical training upon entrance into the university helps students recognize and keep in mind the importance and the challenge of community health care. This is expected to motivate students to pursue the subject. Furthermore, the joint program allows students to meet those who share the same interest in community health, leading to reinforcement of their interest.

3.1.4 Coping with Current Issues

A shortage of doctors and other health professionals in the prefecture is a serious problem in Hokkaido, particularly in rural areas. Hopefully, the above-mentioned initiatives will result in reducing the workload of health professionals in those areas by fostering the students' appreciation of and commitment to community health care. This, in turn, will assist the university in maintaining high recruitment and retention rates of health professionals in Hokkaido.

Table 2. Interprofessional community training programs of the university

School year	Learning task	Content
1	Formation of appreciation for community health and partners	Communications training Group study for understanding diverse professions Study for understanding community profile and characteristics
2	Identification of issues	Dialogue with and understanding of community people Discussion with community health personnel Discussion with administration officer Group study on health issues in the community
3	Consideration of assistance measures	Support for alleviating health problems of individual, family, and groups Design of assistance measures for health promotion Discussion on administration issues in community health
4	Presentation of results	Poster presentation, reporting to parties concerned inside and outside the school, Best Portfolio and Poster Award

3.2 Management Structure of the Programs

3.2.1 Joint Curriculum Across Schools (Team-based Residential Community Internship)

The team-based residential community internship was the first joint curriculum of the two schools, with the President as the Executive Director and the Dean of the School of Health Science as the Program Manager. The Planning and Evaluation Core Group, which plays a central role in program management, consisted of the academic staff of the two schools (four staff members each); this Core Group plans, implements, and evaluates the program. Later, the Program Support Group, consisting of 11 professors from the two schools, was created to play an advisory role for the Core Group. At a joint meeting, the Core Group presents a program plan to the Support Group for review and discussion and thereafter finalizes it as advised. The academic staff of the Core Group also plays an important role in implementation. They guide students to program sites and facilitate students' active participation in the program. In addition, the university's administration officer, who is familiar with the program sites, helps coordinate the program with health facilities and local governments. Thus, the entire university commits itself to the program (Fig. 5).

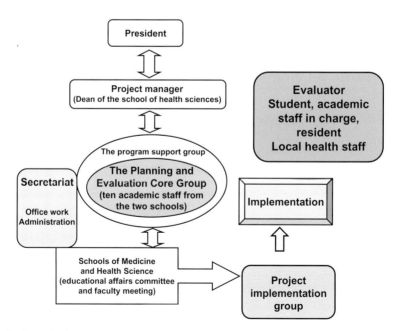

Fig. 5. Organization

3.2.2 Plan for Upgrading the Program to the Joint Regular Curriculum and Creating a Joint Seminar for Community Health Care

The program management structure includes the Core Group, which plays a central role in program management, and the Sub-Group, consisting of related academic staff. The management proposes new curricula, reviews existing ones in pursuit of joint curricula for the two schools, and improves the team-based residential community health care internship. It is important to coordinate annual and monthly schedules of the management groups and post an administration officer to liaise with academic staff for smooth program implementation.

4 IPE Characteristics: Advantages and Originality

In the vast geographical area of Hokkaido, maldistribution of medical personnel is responsible for the scarcity of medical services. The university, prioritizing human resource development to support community heath, is implementing various training programs, such as the team-based residential community health internship. This is to enhance students' appreciation of community health care and the team-based collaborative capability that is essential for community health care. Our programs have a strong advantage in that they systematically offer community health training from the outset of the students' education. Indeed, the efforts are beyond just an isolated attempt.

The described education program, of a duration of 3½ years, makes it possible to build up the education programs in a consistent, sustainable manner. Moreover, the program has proven effective in achieving our educational goals.

5 IPE Outcome: Evaluation

5.1 Evaluation of the Programs and Program Effect

The above-mentioned residential community and team-based training programs aim at producing professionals who serve the community. These programs help students increase their interest in community health as professionals through practice training during their initial school years. Furthermore, the residential joint curricula (team-based residential community health care internship) provide students with an opportunity to interact with medical professionals as well as patients and their families. This opens their eyes to disease prevention for residents of the community and to community issues in general. This effect was confirmed by self-assessment questionnaires of students who participated in the joint program (a before-and-after study using a visual analogue scale) (Fig. 6).

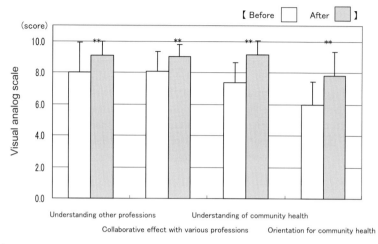

Fig. 6. Team-based residential community internship program: self-evaluation ($n = 34$) before and after the program. **$P < 0.01$, Mann-Whitney U-test

5.2 Evaluation Method and System

Students evaluate residential community training and team-based training programs using a marking sheet. Community health staff, residents, and responsible academic staff, in addition to students, also evaluate the internship program by filling out questionnaires. The university shares the evaluation results with the people involved, learns lessons from the results, and incorporates what it has learned to improve the next training program. For the internship program, a before-and-after study is conducted on students' attitudes toward community health. A survey is done during the preparatory phase and before and after internship program implementation. The results indicate that students gain an enthusiasm in community health and strengthened sensitivity toward it. Proposals are also made, based on the results, to expand and improve the curriculum.

5.3 Program Planning Process

A wide range of individuals are engaged in program planning, management, and evaluation (outputs and general information). The group includes not only students, instructors, and academic staff of the Core Group but also residents, community leaders, and a third party outside the university. Evaluation methods include various questionnaires as described, student presentations, reports, and portfolio evaluation. Students' portfolios are digitized for effective information management, which helps collect, save, share, and analyze information more widely.

Interprofessional Education at Niigata University of Health and Welfare

Implementation of an Integrated General Seminar and Future Prospects

Rieko Oshiki[1], Akira Magara[2], Emiko Hoshino[3], Yasuyuki Nishihara[4], Seiya Masegi[4], Eikichi Watanabe[5], Masato Kaibuchi[6], Yoichi Nagai[6], and Hideaki E. Takahashi[7]

Summary

Since its establishment, Niigata University of Health and Welfare has been actively involved in interprofessional education: Basic Seminars I and II (introductory programs for first-year students); basic lectures on health care and welfare (a core curriculum for students in all departments); and the Integrated General Seminar for fourth-year students. We herein report the significance of the program and the educational achievements. The Integrated General Seminar was held in 2004 on a

---

[1]Department of Physiotherapy, Faculty of Medical Technology, Niigata University of Health and Welfare, Niigata, Japan
[2]Department of Prosthetics & Orthotics and Assistive Technology, Faculty of Medical Technology, Niigata University of Health and Welfare, Niigata, Japan
[3]Department of Social Welfare, Faculty of Social Welfare, Niigata University of Health and Welfare, Niigata, Japan
[4]Department of Health and Sports, Faculty of Health Sciences, Niigata University of Health and Welfare, Niigata, Japan
[5]Department of Health and Nutrition, Faculty of Health Sciences, Niigata University of Health and Welfare, Niigata, Japan
[6]Department of Occupational Therapy, Faculty of Medical Technology, Niigata University of Health and Welfare, Niigata, Japan
[7]Niigata University of Health and Welfare, 1398 Shimamicho, Kita-ku, Niigata 950-3198, Japan
Tel. +81-25-257-4455; Fax +81-25-257-4456
e-mail: takahasi@nuhw.ac.jp

Correspondence to: H.E. Takahashi

trial basis for the first fourth-year students and formally introduced in 2008. The number of students who attend the Integrated General Seminar is increasing: from 70 students in 2007 to 100 students in 2008. The seminar encourages students to develop specialized skills while recognizing the expertise of those from other departments and learning from them; they also learn to design and implement care and assessment plans for patients using disease and lifestyle models. Students learn the basic methods and procedures necessary to provide patients with care in collaboration with other health care professionals through simulations of multidisciplinary care.

Key words Interprofessional education · Interprofessional work · Health care and welfare

1 Profile and Mission of the University

Since the end of World War II, Japan has seen a steady increase in the average life expectancy, with priority being given to longevity. During the 1980s, however, quality of life (QOL) started to attract public attention. As the Japanese population ages during the 21st century, it is essential to provide consistent, integrated health care and welfare services. Today's advanced, sophisticated, specialized medical services are provided by a variety of health care professionals; and it is becoming necessary to train a large number of welfare specialists to address the aging population. In April 2001, Niigata University of Health and Welfare was established to meet these demands in the society.

The mission of the university is to train excellent quality of life (QOL) supporters. Thus, the school aims to train professionals who will help promote the QOL of care recipients, patients, and the elderly.[1] Qualities required for the QOL supporter are compassion, brightness, enthusiasm, creativity, and cooperative skills.

With the purpose of enhancing close collaboration among medical and welfare professionals, the university established departments related to medical technology, social welfare, and nutrition. Until 2004, the university consisted of two faculties (Medical Technology and Social Welfare) and five departments. The Medical Technology Faculty included the following departments: Physical Therapy; Occupational Therapy; Speech, Language, and Hearing Sciences; and Health and Nutrition. The Social Welfare Faculty included the Department of Social Welfare. As of 2009, the university has three faculties and eight departments, with the Departments of Health and Sports (2005), Nursing (2006), and Prosthetics & Orthotics and Assistive Technology (2007) being established. The university was reorganized into three faculties in 2007, when the Faculty of Health Sciences, being added, included the Departments of Health and Nutrition, Health and Sports, and Nursing. The master's program of the Graduate School of Health and Welfare was started in 2005 and the doctoral program in 2007.

Since its establishment, Niigata University of Health and Welfare, designed to train specialists with advanced expertise who will closely cooperate with other health care and welfare professionals, has provided interprofessional education (IPE) for undergraduate and graduate students.[2] In this chapter, we summarize its curriculum design and implementation as well as that of the Integrated General Seminar for fourth-year students.

2 Core Curriculum and Interprofessional Education

Preparation for establishing the university started in 1999, and in 2000 a preparatory office, consisting of staff members and one person from each of the departments, was organized. This developed into the preparatory foundation. At the initial stage of IPE, all academic staff of the university participated in discussions to plan and develop programs. Basic Seminar I, held during the first semester of the first academic year, placed emphasis on communication between instructors and students (≤10 students). Basic Seminar II, held during the second semester of the first year, was designed to allow students to learn the importance of interprofessional activities. Other programs, part of the core curriculum, included 19 mandatory and selective subjects for first- to fourth-year students in all departments (Fig. 1).

The curriculum is revised every 4 years. In 2003, a curriculum plan for 2005 to 2008, including the Integrated General Seminar for fourth-year students, was developed. The Integrated General Seminar, initiated in 2004, is designed to encourage students to learn about the expertise and characteristics of other care professionals

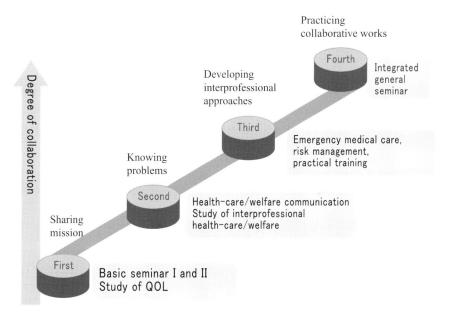

Fig. 1. Educational goals of interprofessional education and the corresponding subjects for each academic year (*First, Second, Third, Fourth*) during 2005–2008. The degree of collaboration is also indicated. *QOL*, quality of life

while developing their own specialized knowledge by creating assessment/support plans and experiencing simulated multidisciplinary care. It is here that they can acquire the basic cooperative skills necessary to provide support and care for patients.

The Integrated General Seminar, included in the 2005 revised curriculum, was scheduled to start in 2008. However, we implemented it earlier than the original schedule, during 2004–2007, because we wanted to introduce it—an unprecedented attempt—in an effective, efficient way. Figure 1 shows the academic subjects related to interprofessional education and the goals for each school year: addressing the mission (during the first year); learning about the problems to be faced (during the second year); developing interprofessional approaches (during the third year); and practicing collaborative skills (during the fourth year).[2]

3 Implementation of the Integrated General Seminar

In 2004, a patient with quadriplegia participated as a volunteer in the seminar held under the theme: "Support for the disabled in the community." The seminar was provided in the form of lectures twice a week over a period of 7 weeks, in which students assessed disabled people regarding their physical functioning in daily life and then held case conferences to develop care plans. Two students and one instructor from each of the Departments of Physical Therapy (PT), Occupational Therapy (OT), Speech Therapy (ST), Health and Nutrition (HN), and Social Welfare (SW) participated.[3]

In 2005, the seminar was held for three groups of students at a comprehensive community sports club and a nursing care facility for the elderly under two themes. For the theme 1 seminar, we recruited participants from community residents instead of simulated patients, and students held discussions to develop specific programs for individual residents based on their physical and nutritional status. For the theme 2 seminar, students conducted a professional assessment of care facility residents with different social backgrounds and designed appropriate plans based on conducting rounds to help them return to their homes.

In 2006, we introduced case studies of amyotrophic lateral sclerosis (ALS) patients based on scenarios. Watching documentary video programs, students from multidisciplinary areas held discussions to identify patients' needs, share information with each other, and develop appropriate support plans. Setting specific plans and academic goals for each session, we held the seminar once a week over a period of 7 weeks, and two students from each of the PT, OT, ST, HN, and SW departments (10 students total) and nine instructors from the PT, OT, ST, HN, HS (Health and Sports), and SW departments participated.

In 2007, a total of 90 students and 19 instructors from six departments participated in the seminar. Using examples of six disease models (four types), as shown in Table 1, student groups assessed the conditions of patients and planned and developed care plans.

Table 1. Themes, subjects, and types of model of the Integrated General Seminar from 2004 to 2008

Year	Theme	Subject model	Type of model
2004	Designing home care plans for a patient with quadriplegia due to cervical cord injury	Physical disability	Actual patient
2005	1. Participation in health management for community residents	Health promotion	Actual patients
	2. Suggestions of home care plans for the elderly after discharge from nursing care facilities	Physical disability	Actual patients
2006	1. Designing home care plans for an ALS patient	Medical care	Patients on video
2007	1. Designing home care plans for patients with stroke sequelae	Physical disability	Patients on video
	2. Assessment of ALS patients and support for home living	Medical care	Patients on video
	3. Patients with spastic cerebral paralysis	Developmental disorders	Actual patients
	4. Support for athletes with sport-related joint injury	Sports disorders	Actual patients
	5. Lifestyle management for patients with possible metabolic syndrome	Health promotion	Simulated patients
2008	1. Home care for patients with cerebrovascular disorders	Physical disability	Simulated cases
	2. Support for a male patient with cerebellar infarction/his participation in social activities	Medical care	Patients on video
	3. Support for patients with spastic cerebral palsy	Developmental disorders	Actual patients
	4. Support for athletes with sport-related injuries	Sports injuries	Actual patients
	5. Advice for patients with (possible) metabolic syndrome	Health promotion	Simulated patients
	6. Lives of the elderly with diabetes	Medical care	Patients on video

ALS, amyotrophic lateral sclerosis

In 2008, the Integrated General Seminar was adopted as a regular selective subject (for one academic credit). Under the guidance of 21 instructors, 75 students in 10 groups examined the examples of six disease models (four types), shown in Table 1. We also successfully introduced some new approaches, including a simulation study of community support for stroke patients and discussions on the web (e.g., opinion exchange with the President of the Onomichi Medical Association, Hiroshima). Significant findings were obtained by studying the approaches of Onomichi in Hiroshima, because the city, with its high aging rate, is known for its advanced approaches, such as community networks between health care and welfare professionals, which are supported by family physicians from Onomichi Medical Association (Professor Katayama).

4 Evaluation of the 2008 Integrated General Seminar

In 2008, we conducted a questionnaire survey of students to evaluate the integrated general seminar prior to the orientation meeting for the seminar (the presurvey) and following general presentations (the postsurvey). The group survey method was employed, and the number of valid responses was 59 (response rate 78.7%). Using t-tests, we compared the results of the two surveys.

Question 1 was "Can you explain your specialty to students in other departments?" We assessed the students' understanding of their future professions on a five-grade scale. The average ± SD was 2.70 ± 0.63 for the presurvey and 3.50 ± 0.66 for the postsurvey, with differences being significant at the 5% level (the 5% level was applied for all comparisons). It is assumed that attending the Integrated General Seminar enhanced their understanding of their future professions.

Question 2 asked students about their knowledge of the future professions of those in other departments. Because we asked students only about members in the group to which they belonged, there were differences in the types and number of departments in each response. Therefore, the mean score of all respondents was interpreted as their "understanding of other professions." The average ± SD was 2.16 ± 0.72 for the presurvey and 3.29 ± 0.49 for the postsurvey. The significant difference between the two surveys demonstrated that attending the Integrated General Seminar enhanced their understanding of the future professions of students in other departments.

Question 3 asked students about their understanding and knowledge of the subjects on which they were learning. The average ± SD was 2.46 ± 0.79 for the presurvey and 3.83 ± 0.57 for the postsurvey. The significant difference between the two surveys demonstrated that what they learned from the Seminar effectively improved their understanding and knowledge of research subjects.

Question 4 asked students about their understanding and knowledge of the subjects on which other groups were working. To calculate the mean score, the score for their own group was deducted from those of each student. The average ± SD was 2.01 ± 0.56 for the presurvey and 2.98 ± 0.50 for the postsurvey. The significant difference between the two surveys demonstrated that attending the Integrated General Seminar increased students' interest in research subjects on which the other groups were working as well as their motivation for learning in general presentations.

Question 5 asked students about their recognition of the significance and importance of addressing research subjects in groups. The average ± SD was 4.59 ± 0.58 in the presurvey and 4.92 ± 0.32 in the postsurvey. The significant

Table 2. Self-assessment by students before and after the Integrated General Seminar: 2008

Assessments by students	Before the seminar	After the seminar	P
Recognition of one's own specialty	2.70 ± 0.63	3.50 ± 0.66	<0.001
Recognition of other specialties	2.16 ± 0.72	3.29 ± 0.49	<0.001
Understanding the case in one's own group	2.46 ± 0.79	3.83 ± 0.57	<0.001
Understanding the case of other groups	2.01 ± 0.56	2.98 ± 0.50	<0.001
Recognition of the importance of IPW	4.59 ± 0.58	4.92 ± 0.32	<0.001
Predictive behavior regarding IPW	4.41 ± 0.79	4.50 ± 0.87	0.594

Results are the average ± SD
IPW, interprofessional work

difference between the two surveys demonstrated that attending the Integrated General Seminar further improved their recognition of the importance of teamwork.

Question 6 asked students about the possibility of working with other professionals. The average ± SD was 4.41 ± 0.79 for the presurvey and 4.50 ± 0.87 for the postsurvey. No significant difference was observed, which suggested that attending the Integrated General Seminar did not affect students' professional awareness of future professions.

Because the Integrated General Seminar held in 2008 improved students' understanding of research subjects in which both they and other groups were involved and increased their awareness of future professions, we concluded that its educational effects had been proven (Table 2).

5 Future Perspectives for 2009 and Beyond

In the revised 2009 curriculum, interprofessional programs were introduced for all students (from the first year through the fourth year). During the Integrated General Seminar, the fourth-year students review what they have learned from health care and welfare lectures and training. Japan has the fastest aging society worldwide and the largest number of patients in need of nursing care due to stroke, followed by dementia, bone fractures, and joint diseases. The Integrated General Seminar covers these disorders and lifestyle-related diseases such as hypertension and diabetes, which are causes of stroke.

The university now has eight departments, and there are more than 650 students in each grade. It is difficult to obtain case examples from approximately 100 groups, including community health care and welfare facilities. In 2008, we held web discussions with the city of Onomichi in Hiroshima Prefecture for this seminar. We are determined to make further efforts and develop an IPE system that employs simulation examples, based on information and communication technologies (ICT), for medical and welfare-focused students.

6 Discussion

Because health care workers must hold discussions with other medical professionals to decide the best care plan for patients regarding treatment options and how to maintain their health, prevent diseases, or support their independent living, students need to develop skills to express their thoughts, listen to others, and recognize and summarize differences in their opinions and viewpoints. The Integrated General Seminar, in a sense, comprises pre-on-the-job-training for multidisciplinary groups, in which students from different departments present their views, develop specialized skills, and learn to recognize the viewpoints of others while debating and consolidating what they have learned. At this significant seminar, students acquire advanced knowledge, deep insights, cooperation skills, and other basic skills required of medical and welfare specialists as well as members of society. The Integrated General Seminar is designed to provide value-added education not provided in any other training sessions organized by individual departments.

The health outcomes of treatment for diseases vary depending on the prefecture in Japan. Therefore, interprofessional education should correspond with the need for interprofessional work in active practice. Furthermore, professionals should be aware of local differences and needs to extend a healthy life expectancy.[4]

7 Conclusion

For the 8 years since 2001 (plus 1 year laying the preparatory foundation), Niigata University of Health and Welfare has provided interprofessional education for health care and welfare-focused students. We report the results of educational projects implemented for students during each academic year. These educational activities were implemented through the collaboration of all of the academic and administrative staff, with their enthusiasm and recognition of the significance of interprofessional education. We are determined to further promote our collaborative efforts. Our graduates will put what they have learned from interprofessional education into practice and promote favorable outcomes for care recipients, patients, and the disabled and elderly. Emulating the practice of IPE developed in the United Kingdom,[5] some universities in Japan are taking new approaches to implement cooperative education, including the establishment of the Japan Association for Interprofessional Education. Although favorable results have been obtained from cooperation among medical professionals, collaboration between health care and welfare has just started. Further efforts should be made to promote and implement interprofessional education in this area.

References

1. Takahashi HE (2001) Establishment of Niigata University of Health and Welfare. Niigata J Health Welfare 1:2–5
2. Takahashi HE (2006) The practice of interprofessional education and its prospect at Niigata University of Health and Welfare Niigata J Health Welfare 6:112–116
3. Makita M, Murayama N, Nishihara Y, et al (2006) Trial of a new collaborative education system: summary of a two-year trial of comprehensive seminars. Niigata J Health Welfare 6:120–125
4. Takahashi HE (2007) Interprofessional education needs to correspond with the necessity of interprofessional work in health-care and welfare in Japan. Niigata J Health Welfare 7:1–8
5. Barr H (2008) Interprofessional education: from rhetoric to reality. Niigata J Health Welfare 8:90–98

Interprofessional Education Program of the University of Tsukuba: A Program to Develop Interprofessional Competence

Takami Maeno[1], Ayumi Takayashiki[1], Tetsuhiro Maeno[1], Tokie Anme[2], Akira Hara[1], Yuka Saeki[2], Osamu Urayama[3], and Fujio Otsuka[1]

Summary

This experience-based educational program is designed to train health professionals to provide a high level of interprofessional care. The program emphasizes practical learning and students' experience in more than 10 health care professions in clinical settings. Introduced in 2004, the program has been administered jointly by three schools (Medicine, Nursing, and Medical Sciences) of the University of Tsukuba. The program features simulated care conferences and discussions in small groups consisting of students from the three schools. The program also provides opportunities for students to learn the viewpoints of patients and a variety of health professionals as well as the cooperative skills and partnerships required for interprofessional work. The program encourages students to understand the importance of cooperation among health professionals, to understand their

---

[1] School of Medicine, School of Medicine and Medical Sciences, University of Tsukuba, 1-1-1 Tennodai, Tsukuba 305-8575, Japan
Tel. +81-29-853-3311; Fax +81-29-853-3002
e-mail: takami-m@md.tsukuba.ac.jp
[2] School of Nursing, School of Medicine and Medical Sciences, University of Tsukuba, Tsukuba, Japan
[3] School of Medical Sciences, School of Medicine and Medical Sciences, University of Tsukuba, Tsukuba, Japan

Correspondence to: T. Maeno

All authors belong to the Committee on Interprofessional Education of the School of Medicine and Medical Sciences.

expertise, and to learn how to develop the relationships necessary for providing interprofessional care.

Key words Interprofessional work · Experience-based educational program · Collaboration · Partnership

1 Profile and Mission of the University of Tsukuba

Since its establishment in 1973, the University of Tsukuba has taken various pioneering approaches based on innovative concepts, moving beyond the conventional Japanese education systems. One example is our educational organization consisting of schools and colleges, instead of faculties and departments. The schools are designed to meet the university's educational goals and are responsible for their students' comprehensive education. The colleges belonging to the various schools are responsible for their students' basic education. In 2007, to improve the curricula, we reorganized the educational structure into nine schools and 23 colleges (Table 1). This organizational system has two main features: The schools and colleges cultivate each student's talents in a broad range of academic fields by encouraging academic endeavors with advisors from various disciplines. The schools and colleges also strive to go beyond the existing aca-

Table 1. Undergraduate Courses

School	Colleges
School of Humanities and Culture	College of Humanities
	College of Comparative Culture
	College of Japanese Language and Culture
School of Social and International Studies	College of Social Sciences
	College of International Studies
School of Human Sciences	College of Education
	College of Psychology
	College of Disability Sciences
School of Life and Environmental Sciences	College of Biological Sciences
	College of Agro-Biological Resource Sciences
	College of Geoscience
School of Sciences and Engineering	College of Mathematics
	College of Physics
	College of Chemistry
	College of Engineering Sciences
	College of Policy and Planning Sciences
School of Informatics	College of Information Science
	College of Media Arts, Science, and Technology
	College of Knowledge and Library Sciences
School of Medicine and Medical Sciences	School of Medicine
	School of Nursing
	School of Medical Sciences
School of Health and Physical Education	
School of Art and Design	

demic system to create the educational foundation needed for each student's future development.

The School of Medicine and Medical Sciences consists of the School of Medicine, the School of Nursing, and the School of Medical Sciences. The three schools' common goal is to train health professionals to develop not only medical expertise but also the communication skills required for a holistic approach.

2 Background and Goals of the Interprofessional Education Program

The aging population of Japan combined with a declining birth rate and other social changes have recently led to substantial changes in medical needs. Physicians are being asked not only to cure disease with drugs and surgery to play other, additional roles. They are expected to take a holistic approach to lifestyle-related disease, mental illnesses, and other health problems and to provide quality care for patients while paying attention to their social and psychological backgrounds.

In this social context, it is difficult for physicians to provide comprehensive and composite health services according to diversified patient needs unless they closely cooperate with other health care professionals—including nurses and social workers—and organize interprofessional care teams. However, today's health care education of medical knowledge and techniques is based on the viewpoint of only physicians. In Japan, there have been few structured interprofessional education (IPE) programs to help students recognize the expertise of other health professionals and the importance of close collaboration with them, as well as to learn skills required for interprofessional care.

This project aims to implement a structured IPE program to train health professionals in the following abilities and practical skills necessary to provide interprofessional care.

- Humanitarianism and communication skills required for health professionals
- Interdisciplinary, comprehensive approaches to health problems from the standpoint of a patient
- Deep understanding of other health care professions
- Cooperative skills necessary for a member of an interprofessional care team

3 Educational Content of the IPE Program

3.1 New Integrated Curriculum of the School of Medicine

Upon the establishment of the University of Tsukuba, the School of Medicine introduced an advanced medical education curriculum earlier than any other

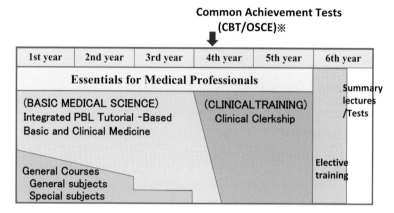

Fig. 1. Curriculum of the School of Medicine. *Common achievement tests for medical and dental students prior to a clinical clerkship. *CBT*, computer-based testing; *OSCE*, objective structured clinical examination; *PBL*, problem-based learning

medical school in Japan. This curriculum was called the Tsukuba Method, and it has achieved satisfactory results. In 2004, in response to rapid changes in today's medical circumstances and social needs, the school introduced a new integrated curriculum, which places emphasis on the "essentials for medical professionals," problem-based learning (PBL) tutorials, and clinical clerkships (Fig. 1).

A major feature of the curriculum is the Essentials for Medical Professionals course provided through the first to fifth academic years, which teaches students to learn essential clinical skills beyond the categories of organs and symptoms. The Essentials for Medical Professionals course consists of seven units: interprofessional work, the patient–doctor relationship, primary health care, medical safety, health promotion, medical ethics, and professionalism.

3.2 Program to Develop Interprofessional Competence

The Program to Develop Interprofessional Competence consists of (1) a medical education curriculum (Fig. 2, right), in which students acquire knowledge and skills as medical doctors, and (2) interprofessional work units in the Essentials for Medical Professionals course (Fig. 2, left), in which students develop interprofessional competence.

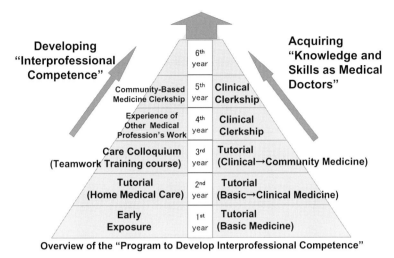

Fig. 2. Overview of the program to develop interprofessional competence

3.2.1 Essentials for Medical Professionals Course: Interprofessional Work Units (Table 2).

In the interprofessional work units, students develop interprofessional competence through practical training. Students are able to experience other (10 or more) medical professions and learn about their expertise and viewpoints—experiences not afforded by lectures. Students come to understand the role of physicians in interprofessional care by reviewing their work from the standpoint of other health professionals.

3.2.1.1 First Year: "Early Exposure"

Various training programs (Figs. 3, 4) to experience health professions are provided during the first academic year, just after entrance to the School of Medicine, with the following objectives.

- Learn communication skills essential for interprofessional care (communication training)
- Understand patients' inconvenience and anxieties (experiencing old age, pregnancy, inpatient experience)
- Understand the roles of many different health professionals in clinical settings from the standpoint of a patient (inpatient experience, hospital ward visit, outpatient escort program)
- Experience the work of different health care professionals to learn their roles (hospital ward visit and community health and welfare institution visit)

Table 2. Interprofessional work units in the Essentials for Medical Professionals course

Program	Purpose	Program content	No. of students	Period	Year of initiation
First year: Essentials for Medical Professionals I (two credits)—early exposure					
Communication training	To learn communication skills necessary to establish relationships with patients and members of the medical team	Interview with simulated patients and group discussions	Four students × 25 groups × 5	Two lessons	2004
Experiencing old age, pregnancy	To learn the importance of daily life care from the standpoints of older adults and pregnant women	Students put on outfits designed to allow the wearer to experience the difficulty with mobility that older adults or pregnant women have. In so doing, they understand the need of such individuals for assistance in everyday life	Ten students × 1 group × 10	Two lessons	2004
Hospital ward visit	To learn the work procedures in a hospital ward while communicating with patients	Helping nurses and nursing assistants in the hospital ward (serving meals and bed making)	Two to three students × 9 groups × 5	Three lessons × 2 days	2004
Inpatient experience	To understand the feelings of inpatients and learn the roles of health professionals in the hospital ward from the standpoint of a patient	Simulated experience of hospitalization in the university hospital (spend one night with other patients)	Ten students × 10 groups	One night (from the evening to the following morning)	2004
Outpatient escort program	To learn the system of a hospital and the roles of various health care professionals in outpatient services from the viewpoint of a patient	Escort outpatients to help them through the procedures (reception, diagnosis, treatment, payment of hospital bills)	Sixteen students × 6 groups × 6 days	1 Day	2004
Community health and welfare institution visit	Experience the work of a variety of care workers in local facilities	Students accompany nurses on home visits or help the staff at homes for the elderly	Two to five students × 9 groups × 3	2 Days	2004

Table 2. (continued)

Program	Purpose	Program content	No. of students	Period	Year of initiation
Second year: Essentials for Medical Professionals II (two credits)—home medical care course					
Home medical care course	To learn the roles of many health professionals in home care settings while paying attention to the feelings of patients and their families	PBL tutorial of patient care and family support using examples of home medical care/participation in lectures by care managers	Eight students × 14 groups	1 Week	2005
Third year: Essentials for Medical Professionals III (two credits)—care colloquium (teamwork training course)					
Care colloquium (teamwork training course)	To learn the importance of interprofessional collaboration to provide quality care	Simulated conference (tutorial) using case scenarios in small interprofessional groups consisting of students of the Schools of Medicine, Nursing, and Medical Sciences	Eight students × 28 groups (including students of the Schools of Nursing and Medical Science)	1 Week	2006
Fourth year: Essentials for Medical Professionals IV (two credits)—experience of other medical profession's work					
Nursing training	To learn the roles of nurses in clinical practice and interprofessional work	Experience the work of ward nurses, including night duties, in the university hospital	Five students × 5 groups × 4	4 Days + 2 nights	1977
Training in the inspection department	To learn the roles of medical technologists in clinical practice and interprofessional care	Experience the work of medical technologists	Twenty-five students × 4 groups	Two lessons × 2 days	1977
Training in the pharmaceutical department	To learn the roles of pharmacists in clinical practice and interprofessional care	Experience the work of pharmacists in the university hospital	Twenty-five students × 4 groups	Two lessons	1995
Fifth year: Essentials for Medical Professionals V (two credits)—community-based medicine clerkship					
Community-based medicine clerkship	To learn how health care/welfare collaboration in community health care settings is different from that in the university hospital	Practical training at local clinics, the homes of patients, and welfare facilities	Five students × 5 groups × 4	2004—1 week 2008—2 to 4 weeks	2004, elective subject 2008, mandatory subject

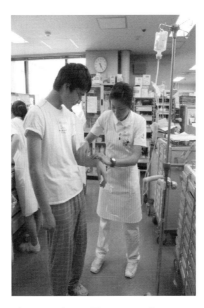

Fig. 3. Early exposure/inpatient experience. The purpose is to promote an understanding of the feelings of inpatients being attached to an intravenous line all night long. In this picture, a nurse is attaching an intravenous tube to the arm of a student

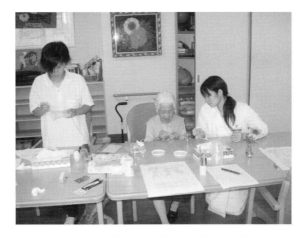

Fig. 4. Early exposure/community health and welfare institution visit. A student is helping a nursing care worker

3.2.1.2 Second Year: Home Medical Care Course

Through case study discussions regarding the care plan for a patient receiving home medical care, students learn the roles of various health care professionals who support patients at home.

3.2.1.3 Third Year: Care Colloquium (Teamwork Training Course)

Introduced in 2006, the Care Colloquium (teamwork training course) is a joint program of the three schools—School of Medicine (100 third-year students), School of Nursing (80 fourth-year students), and School of Medical Sciences (40 fourth-year students)—the objective of which is to help students learn the importance of interprofessional work and collaboration (Figs. 5, 6). Students from the three schools are placed in small groups of seven or eight each to discuss the roles of different health professionals and how they should share patient information and cooperate with each other. Using case scenarios of aging adults in need of community health, terminal, and other interprofessional care, students are encouraged through discussions to promote their understanding of the specific role of various medical professionals and are expected to recognize the importance as well as the difficulties of communicating and sharing information with other care professionals.

The program is managed and implemented by the faculty of the three schools: 4 coordinators (2 faculty members from medicine, 1 from nursing, and 1 from medical sciences), 7 scenario writers (all from nursing), and 28 tutors (3 from medicine, 15 from nursing, and 10 from medical sciences).

3.2.1.4 Fourth Year: Experiencing Other Health Professionals' Work in Tsukuba University Hospital

In the preclinical clerkship (PreCC) program, students experience the work of a nurse, pharmacist, medical technologist, and other specialists in Tsukuba University Hospital. The program is designed to facilitate students' understanding of the roles of nurses and other specialists in clinical practice as well as the expected role

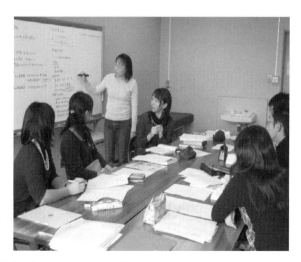

Fig. 5. Care Colloquium (teamwork training course): small-group discussion by students of the three schools

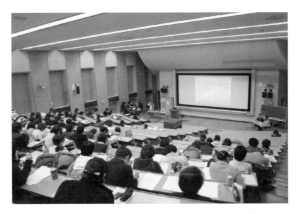

Fig. 6. Care Colloquium (teamwork training program): general presentation meeting

of physicians in interprofessional care from the viewpoint of different health professionals.

3.2.1.5 Fifth Year: Community-based Medicine Clerkship

Students learn the characteristics of interprofessional care provided in the community, including that from local clinics, hospitals, and home care. Students are expected to note differences between care services provided in the community and those provided in university hospitals (e.g., the emphasis of community-based medicine on nursing and welfare care) (Fig. 7).

3.2.2 Interprofessional Education in Other Medical Education Curricula

Students are also encouraged to develop their skills for interprofessional work not only in the interprofessional work unit but also in other courses. They acquire communication and collaborative skills in PBL tutorials during the first to third academic years and develop practical expertise for interprofessional work in clinical clerkships during the fourth and fifth academic years.

3.2.2.1 First to Third Years: Basic Medicine and Preclinical Training Curriculum Based on PBL Tutorial-based Learning

PBL tutorials are implemented in all courses, from basic to clinical medicine. Students obtain health care information from case scenarios in simulated clinical settings where physicians, nurses, and many different health professionals are involved in patient care (Box 1). The PBL tutorial helps students develop communication and relationship skills essential for interprofessional work. Through group discussions, students come to understand a wide range of views and thoughts, and they learn how to organize their ideas and convey them to others.

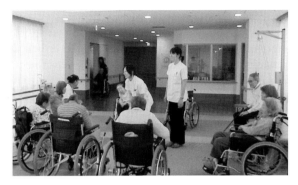

Fig. 7. Community-based medicine clerkship. Exercise techniques are being taught by students to elderly residents in a nursing home

Box 1

Examples of tutorial scenarios
(A scenario for second-year students in the respiratory system course: 2005)

Making rounds, Dr. Mitsui talks to Mr. Sakura, a patient who has just undergone surgery: "You are recovering well, and I know you are walking around well after your surgery." "Well, the nurses told me to walk as much as possible. They said that I should get up and walk to prevent any complications after my operation. It's a bit hard. But, it's important for me to recover, and all the ward staff are very kind and supportive..."

3.2.2.2 Fourth and Fifth Years: Clinical Clerkships

In this course, students are required to attend clinical practice as members of medical teams. To encourage students to communicate more and develop relationships with team members, including nurses and ward clerks, we extended the period of training in a single hospital ward from 2 weeks to 2 months and the total period from 1 year to 1½ years. Students can effectively develop competence for interprofessional work through the clinical clerkships.

4 Characteristics of the IPE Program

4.1 Characteristics of the IPE Program

First, the IPE program places emphasis on practical training rather than on didactic lectures. This is because passive learning such as that which takes place during lectures is inappropriate as a strategy for developing skills for interprofessional work. Few universities in Japan have implemented large-scale, experience-based programs for interprofessional education because of the difficulties encountered when preparing training sites (i.e., coordinating among departments and obtaining support from medical facilities). As a result, most medical students in Japan become doctors without the experience of interacting with other health professionals or understanding their roles. Furthermore, this situation may last throughout their career. In the program at Tsukuba University, students can improve interprofessional competence effectively; for example, students come to understand patients' feelings and thoughts through experiencing an actual patient; and they come to understand the role of various health professionals by experiencing the work of nurses and other health professionals—experiences not acquired from classroom lectures.

Second, the IPE program is implemented from the first to fifth academic years as the core program in the Essentials for Medical Professionals course. Previously, such programs were provided in a complementary manner in the curriculum. Thus, beginning with the time immediately after admission to clinical training in the senior year, students have many opportunities to interact with patients and a variety of health professionals, and they systematically develop competence for interprofessional work.

Third, the program has been planned and implemented through interprofessional collaboration between the schools of Medicine, Nursing, and Medical Sciences. In the Care Colloquium (teamwork training course), medical and other students have discussions with each other, exchanging views and opinions frankly. Upon the organizational reform of the schools and colleges of Tsukuba University in 2007, the former School of Medicine was reorganized into the School of Medicine and Medical Sciences, consisting of three schools: the School of Medicine, the School of Nursing, and the School of Medical Sciences. Since that reorganization, educational cooperation has been enhanced among the schools, and IPE has been given the position of one of the main subjects in the core curriculum of the School of Medicine and Medical Sciences. We are working to further enhance collaboration within the School of Medicine and Medical Sciences and to increase opportunities for students of the Schools of Medicine, Nursing, and Medical Sciences to learn with, from, and about each other to improve collaboration and quality of care.

4.2 Organization of the Program

Because implementation of this program requires a large number of academic staff ("early exposure" is provided by approximately 100 staff) and contact and communication with university hospitals and local facilities, continued support from educational organizations is essential. The IPE program is supported by the Center of Planning and Coordination for Medical Education (PCME). Established to design, implement, and assess medical education programs, the PCME consisted of 15 faculty (3 full-time and 12 part-time) and 19 technical staff as of April 2008. It supports the development of educational materials and preparation of practical training, implements faculty development (FD) projects, evaluates the effectiveness of the school's educational programs, and performs other educational tasks. In 2003, one of PCME's activities was adopted by the Ministry of Education, Culture, Sports, Science, and Technology as "good practice" (GP). By the end of 2007, a total of 90 faculty members of our medical school had participated in FD for curriculum planning, and more than 350 had participated in FD for PBL tutorial training. The IPE program has been implemented with various types of support from the PCME: contact with medical facilities (training sites), assignment of academic staff, the development of educational materials such as case scenarios, and assessment of programs.

To introduce new joint programs through collaboration among the three schools, we established a system designed to plan, implement, and evaluate interprofessional education programs, with support from the PCME. One such effort was the creation of a Committee on Interprofessional Education of the School of Medicine and Medical Sciences, consisting of staff from the university and external specialists.

5 Efficacy of the IPE Program

Students who participated in "early exposure" (during the first year) positively evaluated "outpatient escort training": 86% answered that it was meaningful, and 75% thought that it should be provided annually. Other comments included: "Explanations to the patient by nurses were detailed and understandable." "I was a bit confused at first because I did not know the system in the university hospital. However, as I escorted patients, I started learning work procedures across multiple departments from their point of view." "When patients thanked me, I was very glad that I was of some help to them." Students learned the roles played by various health professionals from the viewpoint of the patients, and the program significantly increased their motivation to become health professionals. All patients who participated in the outpatient escort training program also commented that it was meaningful for students. The community health and welfare institution visit increased students' respect for other medical professionals: "Helping a patient bathe for only 2 hours exhausted me. It was much harder than I had expected. I am impressed with care workers working hard every day."

At the initiation and completion of the Care Colloquium (teamwork training course), we conducted a questionnaire survey to evaluate its educational effectiveness. We revised the questionnaire employed in a previous survey of the IPE program.[1] The questions were intended to reveal the students' understanding of

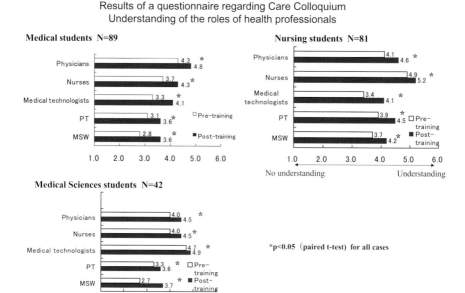

Fig. 8. Results of a questionnaire regarding the Care Colloquium/understanding the roles of medical professionals. Students of the three schools demonstrated an increased understanding of the roles of health professionals after the implementation of Care Colloquium training. *PT*, physiotherapists; *MSW*, medical social workers

the roles of medical professionals, participation in group work, attitudes toward interprofessional care teams, and understanding of the importance of interprofessional collaboration and cooperation. A six-grade Likert scale, between "definitely yes" and "definitely no," was used in the survey. Students of the three schools demonstrated their increased understanding of the roles of health professions after the implementation of the Care Colloquium (Fig. 8). There was also increased awareness of participation in group work and in interprofessional care teams and in their understanding of the importance of interprofessional collaboration and cooperation, which indicates the effectiveness of discussions using scenarios.

About the Care Colloquium, one student reported, "I was surprised at the variety of health professionals involved in patient care. Although it may not be easy for the many different care specialists to cooperate with each other, I learned the importance of interprofessional collaboration through discussions and simulation-based learning." Discussions among students from the three schools raised their awareness of the expertise of other health professionals and the importance of interprofessional cooperation and mutual understanding (Box 2). Academic staff involved in the development of scenarios also evaluated the program positively: "Although we had a hard time preparing scenarios, I was impressed with students' enthusiasm for learning. We will make further efforts to improve the program and its effectiveness."

We also conducted a questionnaire survey to examine the effectiveness of community health care training for fifth-year students. Before and after their training in health clinics we asked the question, "Can you imagine the work of community health professionals, including care managers, helpers, and home visit nurses?" Whereas only 20% of students answered "yes" before the training session, most were able to imagine their work after the session, which indicates an increased understanding of community health care professions (Fig. 9).

Box 2

From a questionnaire survey of students titled "What did you learn from the Care Colloquium?"

- It is difficult to act in the best interests of patients without cooperation from other health professionals. I learned the importance of cooperation within an interprofessional team in providing patients with health care. (Medical student)
- I became more aware of post-treatment patient care. (Medical student)
- To work together with other medical professionals, I need to achieve more professional expertise in my specialty. (Medical student)
- I found it difficult to convey my thoughts to those who have been trained in different fields. (Nursing student)
- I learned the standpoints and roles of other medical professionals. (Medical Sciences student)

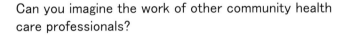

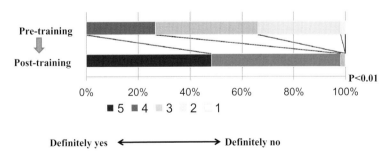

Fig. 9. Results of a questionnaire survey before and after a community-based medicine clerkship

6 Brief Discussion

Although the Program to Develop Interprofessional Competence has achieved significant results, it is centered on simulated care conferences using case scenarios. We are planning to improve the program and place more emphasis on joint training sessions in clinical settings for students throughout the entire School of Medicine and Medical Sciences (all three schools). We will improve our IPE program for medical, nursing, and medical sciences students to learn with, from, and about each other to develop interprofessional competence.

The mission of the School of Medicine and Medical Sciences of the University of Tsukuba is to train medical professionals with these qualities and to develop interprofessional competence required in clinical settings to improve the quality of patient care.

Reference

1. Otsuka M, Maruyama Y, Arai T, et al. (2005) Effects of interprofessional learning in the case study: comparing students before and after interprofessional work in uni-disciplinary and multi-disciplinary groups. The Bulletin of Saitama Prefectural university 7:21–25

Community-Based Interprofessional Education at Saitama Prefectural University

Mariko Otsuka[1], Midori Shimazaki[2], Kazunori Kayaba[3], Takanori Sakada[1], Kazuhiko Hara[4], Masaya Asahi[2], Toshitami Arai[2], Ikuo Murohashi[3], Keiko Yokoyama[1], Naomi Hasegawa[1], Minoru Kawamata[5], Reiko Suzuki[1], Chiyo Fujii[2], Naoko Kunisawa[3], Miyuki Kanemune[1], Noriko Shimasue[2], Hiromi Shinmura[1], Ken Nishihara[4], Kazuhisa Inoue[4], Kumi Ogawa[2], and Rumi Tano[3]

Summary

Saitama Prefectural University (SPU) aims to turn its students into high-quality health and social care professionals who understand the need for working in cooperation with professionals in other disciplines and are competent working with them. SPU offers interprofessional experiences to students to accomplish its stated aims. Based on the principle of interprofessional education, SPU has created an educational framework for achieving collaborative and integrated health and social services. The university provides opportunities from which students can learn, with and about each other beyond the boundaries of their departments and disciplines. In 2005, SPU was selected as one of the universities to be provided with a national

---

[1]Department of Nursing, Saitama Prefectural University School of Health and Social Services, 820 Sannomiya, Koshigaya 343-8540, Japan
Tel./Fax +81-48-973-4151
e-mail: otsuka-mariko@spu.ac.jp
[2]Department of Social Work, Saitama Prefectural University School of Health and Social Services, Koshigaya, Japan
[3]Department of Health Sciences, Saitama Prefectural University School of Health and Social Services, Koshigaya, Japan
[4]Department of Physical Therapy, Saitama Prefectural University School of Health and Social Services, Koshigaya, Japan
[5]Department of Occupational Therapy, Saitama Prefectural University School of Health and Social Services, Koshigaya, Japan

Correspondence to: M. Otsuka

government grant in the Support Program for Contemporary Education Needs. In the study presented, significant differences in learning effects were observed in an interprofessional (IP) study, particularly for the aspects of understanding patients, extracting issues, considering resolutions, understanding other professions' roles, developing perspectives on a team, understanding cooperation and collaboration, and identifying professional roles. The IP study seemed to enable the learning of interprofessional work, which allows students to share objectives in health and social services.

Key words Community-based IPE · Case study · Evaluation

1 Profile and Mission of Saitama Prefectural University

Saitama Prefectural University (SPU), founded in 1999, has five departments—Nursing, Physical Therapy, Occupational Therapy, Social Work, and Health Sciences—in a single faculty named the School of Health and Social Services. The university's mission is to develop well-qualified professionals in the fields of health and social services who can contribute to Japanese society, which has a seriously falling birth rate and a rapidly increasing aging population in the 21st century. The university aims to have the students acquire professional knowledge and skills, engage in interprofessional work well, act according to humanitarian and ethical values, investigate diverse phenomena, develop their critical thinking and global perspectives, and collaborate with communities. Education aiming at the realization of collaborated and integrated services is provided with the support of communities.

2 Background and Goals of the IPE Program

In our aged society, medical and nursing care has become vital, as more elderly people have limited mental and physical function and chronic diseases. The government has emphasized the need to enhance health care activities so as to shorten the period of nursing care for the elderly. Japan has long-term nursing care insurance; and medicine, health care, and social care have gradually become integrated. Furthermore, collaboration among health and social care professionals, staff, and service providers became essential in the areas that require long-term care and have complex, difficult issues. Examples of these areas are care for patients with chronic diseases, terminal care, rehabilitation, measures against child abuse, measures to prevent patients from being permanently bed-ridden, and dementia care.

Saitama Prefectural University aims to turn its students into high-quality health and social care professionals who understand the need for working in cooperation with professionals in other disciplines and are competent when working with them. SPU offers interprofessional experience to the students to accomplish its aims. Based on the principle of interprofessional education (IPE), SPU has created an educational framework for achieving collaborative and integrated health and social services. The university provides opportunities for students to learn from, with, and about each other beyond the boundaries of their departments and disciplines. In 2005, SPU was selected as one of the universities to be awarded a national government grant in the Support Program for Contemporary Education Needs.

SPU faculty members have paid visits, organized by the Centre for the Advancement of Interprofessional Education (CAIPE) in the United Kingdom, to a number of U.K. universities over the years, to observe and discuss how they have developed IPE and to share experiences and exchange ideas. SPU has annually hosted an IPE Conference since 2005, and the conference has had participants from all over Japan. In November 2008, after the IPE conference, the first annual meeting of the Japan Association for Interprofessional Education (JAIPE) was held at SPU.

With cooperation of the Saitama Prefectural Government and its local offices, SPU faculty members visited more than 250 facilities of health and welfare activities throughout Saitama Prefecture from AY 2005–2008. A total of 12 conferences have been organized in 10 Saitama Welfare and Health Administration Office districts. Member facilities include health promotion sections of the local government, hospitals, long-term care facilities, welfare facilities, and nonprofessional offices (NPOs). The conferences aim at promoting interprofessional work within and among facilities and at working with SPU on IPE. The conference is expected to be a bridge between the community and SPU in each region.

3 Educational Content of the IPE Program

SPU has liberal arts courses, general courses, specialized courses, and interprofessional courses. Significantly, the curricula contain interprofessional courses that aim to help students develop a shared knowledge base and a common understanding beyond the boundaries of the departments with the students of other departments so they can work in teams to respond to patients and service users and provide integrated care. These courses are offered with the cooperation of many hospitals and institutions in the prefecture. The university is committed to providing systematic education for collaboration and integration in all departments, aiming at fostering professionals who can work in collaboration and provide integrated services in health and social care.

Interprofessional courses consist of human care, field activities, and interprofessional work (IPW). In addition, students are required to obtain two units or more in other departments.

- The Human Care course, required for all first-year students, helps students learn the common philosophy of care.

- The Field Activities course, an initial interdisciplinary practicum, is required for all the first-year students of the five departments. It provides a basic understanding of person-to-person care, which is the common foundation for health and social services.
- The IPW course is a joint interdisciplinary practicum required for all fourth-year students. All of the students who have completed the major part of their professional practical training form a team and make a care plan for a particular patient or service user, utilizing what they have learned in the university or at the practicum sites.

In the graduate school, students have opportunities to study about interprofessional work, hold discussions, learn with, about, and from one another, and develop their research.

4 Characteristics of the IPE Program

The Human Care course provides students opportunities to consider and learn about care, illnesses, disabilities, aging, mental problems, death, communication, and teamwork. They listen to lectures and have group discussions. The course is taught by the staff of multiple departments.

In the Field Activities course, students work with their peers and faculty members from other departments in actual health and social service provision settings and learn the basics of collaboration and integration through practical, hands-on experience.

SPU has had interprofessional work in practice since 2002. After completing the major part of their professional practical training, fourth-year students from five departments work as a team at a hospital, a social welfare institution, or a comprehensive local support center and make a support plan for a patient or a client through interviews and discussions. When working on a case as a group, the students have discussions presenting different viewpoints with the aim of understanding the person. They exchange opinions, try to understand one another's approaches, and finally arrive at shared common goals and each role for care. At least two facilitators are assigned to each group. One is a professional of the practice institution, and the other is a teacher at SPU. Both participated in facilitator training seminars to learn teaching methods before the practice exercise.

During this process, the students become aware of and can redefine their own professional identities, and they develop a deeper understanding of their own roles as well as those of other professionals. IPW fosters mutual professional understanding.

Promoting interprofessional work in the community through the IPW course and IPW conference discussions, the university teaching staff members have been developing the IPE program.

5 A Study on the IPW Course

Several studies on the evaluation of interprofessional learning have been conducted. This article presents a study which compared students before and after interprofessional work in uni-disciplinary and multi-disciplinary groups.

Objectives

The study was held to clarify IPW course learning effects in an interprofessional practice by comparing it with preplacement effects and postplacement effects of an intraprofessional practice.

Method

The 25 research subjects comprised 5 fourth-year students from each of the four departments in the university (nursing, social work, physiotherapy, occupational therapy) and 5 second- or third-year students from a medical department in a medical college, from whom SPU obtained research cooperation.

To examine the learning effects of IPW, the questionnaires were designed with a framework of four levels of evaluation. The design adopted frameworks at four levels of evaluation for a training program proposed by Kirkpatrick.[4] Among the levels of evaluation shown by Kirkpatrick, "Reaction" (degree of satisfaction in a practice) was excluded because the present study was an experimental practice. "Results" (increase in team power and achievement of objectives for patient supports) was also excluded because the exercise was not aimed to support activity. Therefore, "Learning" and "Behavior" were examined to determine the learning effects of the practices.

At the "Learning" level, we operationalized learning objectives based on the contents of learning in an IPW found in the precedent study. Questions consisted of 14 items on aspects of "understanding of patients," 16 items on "learning outcomes as a team," 10 items on "perception of own professions," 10 items on "understanding other professions' roles," 14 items on "perspectives on a team," and 6 items on "understanding cooperation and collaboration." "Perception of own profession" was based on "identity measurement of professions," proposed by Fujinawa et al.[5] At the "Behavior" level, there were seven question items for "participation in group work." Responses were rated on a scale ranging from "strongly agree" (six points) to "strongly disagree" (one point).

The questionnaires were distributed to the subjects, who were asked to answer the questions and fill in the name of their group and their department but to remain anonymous. The survey was conducted three times: before practices, after a practice with a group of five students within an individual department (henceforth intraprofessional practice), and after a practice with a group of five students including a student from each of four departments in the university and a medical student from a medical college (henceforth IPW). The data from three surveys were set up as three groups.

The statistical software, SPSS11.5 for Windows was used for data analysis. We applied the Friedman test for comparison among three groups of average scores from each question and the Wilcoxon signed-rank test for comparison between two groups.

The fourth-year students in our university were recruited publicly and asked individually to participate in the surveys. The surveys targeted subjects who consented to participate after being given a written explanation of the research. The students from a medical college who participated in a community health care seminar were recruited by lecturers of the community health care center. The same written explanation was given to the subjects before consent was obtained.

Two placements were conducted in two days. An intraprofessional practice conducted on the first day and an IPW on the second day. In other words, the students discussed a clinical case among a group of students from the same department on the first day and among a mixed group of students from other departments on the second day. The group members were randomly selected in a drawing.

Information of the clinical case discussed within the groups was provided by a hospital (at this point, the information was carefully manipulated so as not to identify an individual), and the experimenters, who were lecturers from five departments, based the model case on this information. The model case concerned a 70-year-old woman suffering from cerebral hemorrhage who was transferred to a rehabilitation hospital after acute care was complete. The information at this stage was organized to use for discussion in the intraprofessional practice, and the information at the time of when she was moved to a maintenance ward 6 months later was used for the IPW. Because the same case was discussed at the two practices, it could be expected that the subjects in the IPW would show greater effects in "understandings of patients." Thus, we increased the amount of information and developed a more complicated scheme for the IPW.

The assignments given in both practices were to conduct group workshops in regard to sharing their understanding of the patient, share objectives of patient support, build support plans, discuss what the cooperation and collaboration should be, and then summarize the results in a group report.

Results

As a result, overall self-evaluation by the students was relatively low in understanding the patient. For the items "being able to find ways to collect and analyze the necessary information and resolve issues" and "being able to think about patient support holistically," the average scores increased gradually, and there are significant differences among the three groups. The findings did not show significant differences in understanding the patient's illness and treatment, physical conditions, daily activities, cognitive and emotional stages, life history, current living conditions, family history, or financial condition.

The subjects were asked not only their individual learning outcomes but also learning outcomes as a support team including other members' learning levels. The questions regarding this topic were not given to the subjects prior to the practices but only after the intraprofessional experience and IPW. As shown in Table 2, the average scores significantly increased in 7 of the 16 questions.

On the topic of understanding their own professions, the findings reveal significant differences among the three groups only for the question of "recommending your own profession to junior students." The average score rose after the intraprofessional practice compared with the preplacement score but showed a relative decline after the IPW.

The average scores on understanding other professions were lower in the postplacement survey of the intraprofessional practice than in the preplacement survey but increased after the IPW. Particularly, such a tendency was observed in understanding the roles of nurses and occupational therapists. Given the fact that understanding social workers' roles displayed the lowest average score before the practice, their roles were less likely to be understood, although they gradually came to be understood by other students. The average score of understanding the roles of doctors after the IPW was reduced compared with the preplacement score.

Considering their perspective about being on a team, the average scores in the three surveys reach more than five points, indicating that students participating in the present study were originally well aware of the importance of a team. The average scores for most questions were lower after the intraprofessional practice than before it; the highest scores were in the postplacement survey after the IPW.

The degree of understanding cooperation and collaboration was also high before the practices. They tended to drop after the intraprofessional practice, however, but rose again after the IPW. The average score dropped after the intraprofessional practice especially for the questions "Do cooperation and collaboration with other professions lead to better support within own profession?" "Do cooperation and collaboration allow you to support patients and their family members?" "Do cooperation and collaboration with other professions lead to better reciprocal supports between professions?" Scores rose in the postplacement survey of the IPW but was not enough to reach the score in the preplacement survey.

For the topic "participation in group work," the average score after the intraprofessional practice tended to be lower than the preplacement scores, but the scores rose after the IPW for the questions regarding "communicating efficiently so as to convey own thoughts" and "listening to other members' opinions." The average score for the questions concerning "identifying the professions' roles" gradually increased in a survey after the other, and a significant difference was found between the postplacement scores of the intraprofessional practice and IPW.

Discussion

Comparing the postplacement effects of the intraprofessional practice to those of the IPW, we found a significant increase in average scores for many questions. Overall, the average scores on the topics "understanding of patients" gradually increased in sequence. Because we assumed that a temporal sequence of the practices would possibly influence the degree of the students' understanding of patients, the case discussed in the IPW was developed to be more complex even though it concerned the same patient. With consideration of such conditions, we expected that the students would gain a deeper understanding of the patient during the IPW than during the intraprofessional practice.

Some survey questions did not exhibit significant differences between the postplacement scores of the intraprofessional practice and of the IPW. However, looking at the learning outcomes as a team, there was a significant increase in average scores for many questions. During the IPW the students became more thoughtful when analyzing information, extracting issues, and discussing resolutions, which led us to conclude that more learning effects were observed during the IPW than during the intraprofessional practice.

Another changing pattern of the average scores for some questions was noted where the score dropped on the postplacement survey of the intraprofessional practice compared with the preplacement survey and then rose again on the postplacement survey of the IPW. We considered that this pattern indicated marked learning effects in the IPW. This can be seen, for example, in the results for "understanding of other professions' roles." The students initially thought that they understood other professions before the placements. However, the average score dropped after the intraprofessional practice because the students realized that their understanding of other professions' roles was vague. The students then deepened their understanding of other professions' roles during the IPW by discussing the clinical case with team members from other departments and by learning their roles from them directly.

Among the questions on the topic "understanding of other professions' roles," the only average score that did not reach the preplacement score was for the question regarding "understanding roles of a doctor." This is because the students from the medical department had not yet experienced a clinical placement, and insufficient utilization of their professionalism possibly influenced the results. Therefore, it is suggested that learning effects increase if the students from each profession conduct a practice after finishing their clinical placements, a time when they could utilize their professionalism.

On the topic "perspectives on a team," the average scores tended to drop after the intraprofessional practice but rose again after the IPW. We assumed that the team members at the intraprofessional practice felt an easiness derived from their confidence of being able to understand each other without sufficient communication because they normally study together in the same department and the pressure to understand other team members was low. In contrast, the students were aware of playing their professional roles during the IPW, where other professions were involved. They placed importance on communicating with each other to become acquainted with other members in order to support their patients. Such awareness affected attitudes toward participation in group work. In addition, efforts to become familiar with each other were required because of the unfamiliar medical students from a different university. Therefore, we believe that experiencing and understanding the process of forming a team brought the average score up.

A similar tendency was observed for the topic "participation in group work," where the average scores dropped after the intraprofessional practice and rose after the IPW. Particularly, there was a significant difference between the intraprofessional and IPW for the question regarding "identifying professional roles." With the additional effects of the temporal sequence of the practices as a learning method, the group work in which students from five different departments were involved was better at identifying the roles of each profession.

Given the high average scores on the topic "understanding of cooperation and collaboration," it can be assumed that the groups consisted of students with high awareness of cooperation and collaboration. In the questions that examined the aspect of "integration of professional support," the average scores dropped in the survey after the intraprofessional practice. The score increased after the IPW did not reach the scores in the preplacement survey. This can be attributed to the fact that the discussed case was a model case and the practices were conducted on our campus. As a consequence, the students were unable to realize the discussed results by applying them to the actual patient. The nature of cooperation and collaboration provides supportive activities with patient-oriented and patient-centered approaches. Thus, the practices without the actual patient prevented the students from realizing such elements. It is suggested that IPE requires training methodology that allows actual clinical practice as well as relationships with patients.

More significant differences of learning effects were observed during IPW than with intraprofessional practice, particularly in the aspects of "understanding patients," "extracting issues," "considering resolutions," "understanding other professions' roles," "developing perspectives on a team," and "understanding cooperation and collaboration." Moreover, in the aspect of "participation in group work," the IPW provided greater significance in respect to "identifying professional roles" than did the intraprofessional practice. The IPW seemed to yield learning effects, as it allows students to share objectives for supporting the patient, and it provides collaboration with other professions.

References

1. Otsuka M, Shimazaki M, Oshima N (2004) The present and prospect of interprofessional education: focus on examples of education in United Kingdom and Japan. Quality Nurs 10:6–12
2. Hirata M, Otsuka M, Oshima N, et al (2002) Attempt of clinical education with cooperation and collaboration as a health care team. Saitama Prefect Univ Collected Papers 14:145–150

3. Otsuka M, Maruyama Y, Hirata M (2004) Learning from cooperation of various professions in a clinical practice with in cooperation among four departments: from attempts in fundamental nursing education. Excerpts from the 24th Research Conference of the Japan Academy of Nursing Science, p 449
4. Kirkpatrick DI (1967) Evaluation of training. In: Craig R, Bittel I (eds) Training and development handbook. NewYork: McGraw-Hill
5. Fujinawa S, Mizuno T, Taniai Y, et al (2000) Analyses of survey about students' identity of own profession: pilot study for development of exercise books in a clinical practice (the first report). Saitama Prefect Univ Collected Papers 2:155–160

Jikei University School of Medicine: An Interprofessional Medical Education Program

Osamu Fukushima

Summary

Health care is a patient-centered team approach supported not only by doctors and nurses but also by a wide range of health professionals. The teamwork approach, however, is possible only when team members understand the beliefs, attitudes, perceptions, and values of the other team members. Therefore, the Jikei University School of Medicine started an Interprofessional Education (IPE) program in 1989 wherein students learn to work in teams. Practically speaking, under the IPE program students participate in a multidisciplinary workplace, take some responsibility, assist leaders and staff, and eventually learn the beliefs, attitudes, perceptions, and values of their respective professions. This exercise enables students to acquire the ability to understand others and to work in teams. IPE is a scholastic good practice to establish collaborative thinking and behavior for effective teamwork among students and help their development as professionals. It is important in an intelligent society to prepare students who can work together with various professionals. This ability is necessary in all professions, in addition to the health professions. Thus, Jikei University advocates the importance of IPE as a model of good professional education practice.

Key words Medical education · Work place · Patient safety · Community · Reflective practice

---

Center for Medical Education, Jikei University School of Medicine, 3-25-8 Nishi-Shimbashi, Minato-ku, Tokyo 105-8461, Japan
Tel. +81-3-343-1111; Fax +81-3-5400-1274
e-mail: fukushima@jikei.ac.jp

Correspondence to: O. Fukushima

1 Profile of the University

The Jikei University School of Medicine is a private medical college that has the longest history in Japan; it was founded by Kanehiro Takaki in 1881. Takaki, a graduate of St. Thomas' Medical School in the United Kingdom, founded the Jikei University after his homecoming. He made efforts to introduce and expand the use of the British-type patient-centered medicine in Japan, despite the fact that German research-oriented medicine was prevalent at that time in Japan. Furthermore, impressed by the Nightingale Training School associated with the St. Thomas Hospital, he founded a nursing education institution in 1885, the first of its kind in Japan. Takaki pointed out the importance of team medicine, which he expressed as "doctors and nurses form two pillars." To reflect this philosophy, the Jikei University established the first Department of Nursing, Faculty of Medicine. This organizational structure has enabled the university to offer education in the health professions that includes medicine and nursing under one umbrella (Faculty of Medicine).

The university has embodied the motto of the school, "Do not see the disease; see the patient," as indicated by Takaki. Hence, we have implemented the following programs in health professions education.

- Fiscal year (FY) 2003: a distinctive university educational program supported by the Ministry of Education, Culture, Sports, Sciences, and Technology (MEXT)—an evaluation system of health professions education
- FY2005: A distinctive university educational program supported by the MEXT—an IPE program for undergraduate medical nursing education
- FY2006: a distinctive university educational program to support social needs by the MEXT—an e-learning system for undergraduate students and health care professionals in the community"
- FY2007: a distinctive university educational program supported by the MEXT—promoting community-based medical education for undergraduate medical and nursing students and supporting continuing professional development for health care providers in the community"
- FY2007: high-quality human resource development for health in response to social needs by the MEXT—a program that fosters clinical research for young community doctors
- FY2008: a strategic intercollegiate program by the MEXT—development of an undergraduate medical education curriculum and provision of continuing professional education for health care providers in the community by four medical schools in Tokyo"

Among other things, the IPE program is a key program wherein a wide range of professions contribute to educating medical and nursing students. The program enables students to appreciate the specific culture of different professions by letting students go into the multidisciplinary workplace, work in teams with various professionals, and learn other professions' cultures—their beliefs, attitudes, perceptions, and values. Health care professionals are expected to be able to learn from others. The ability to learn from other professionals helps develop their teamwork capacity as well as their ability to care for patients who have varying values. The program is scholarly and teaches good practice, reflecting the founder's two mottos: "Doctors and nurses form two pillars" and "Do not see the disease; see the patient."

2 Background and Goals of the Program

Traditional medical and nursing education is a uniprofessional endeavor where doctors teach medical students and nurses teach nursing students. However, doctors and nurses are professionals who each hold their own sense of values and culture. Thus, educating medical students only by doctors would result in imprinting only doctors' sense of values on the students. This phenomenon can be a "hidden curriculum," widely seen in professional education beyond the medical field.

One of the founder's mottos is, "Do not see the disease; see the patient." "Seeing" the patient presupposes an understanding that patients have different cultures and lifestyles. Hence, students are requested to grow enough to understand others. In addition, the message of Kanehiro Takaki at the foundation of the first nursing school in 1885, "Doctors and nurses form two pillars," could be translated now into, "Health care is conducted by a team participated in by a variety of health professionals." Thus, Jikei University started thinking about how to prepare undergraduate students to become professionals who understand others and work in teams with other professionals of different cultures. Eventually, in 1989, the university started the IPE program as a way to achieve this purpose. In 1989, the university introduced the subject "the experience of the nursing care program" during the fourth year of the undergraduate medical program in which nurses teach medical students. In 1992, the university established the Department of Nursing, Faculty of Medicine and created subjects common to medical and nursing students. This arrangement has made available a joint learning opportunity between medical and nursing students. The Nursing Department, since its establishment, has implemented subjects wherein professionals other than nurses teach nursing students, such as the following.

- Nursing care for the elderly during the third year of the nursing program
- Nursing care for maternity
- Nursing care for children in practice
- Nursing care for children in hospital
- Nursing care in the community

Teachers include care workers, welfare counselors, child care workers, midwives in the community, and so on.

The university introduced systematic IPE programs in 1996, listed blow, on the occasion of a comprehensive curriculum reform of the Department of Medicine. This was done in a way to advance the initiatives of the Nursing Department.

- Community service program that addresses problems of the handicapped during the first year of the medical curriculum. This is a mandatory subject (one credit) where all first-year medical students are sent to welfare institutions in the community for the duration of 1 week and work there with the staff for service users. The students get instructions and advice on the job directly from the staff, which includes care workers, welfare counselors, and volunteers.
- Program of care for severely handicapped children and incurable patients during the second year of the medical curriculum. This is an elective subject (one credit) where students are sent to health facilities of their choice, such as a hospital for severely handicapped children or a hospice, for 1 week. Students get on-the-job training under the supervision of the facility's staff, which include but are not limited to child welfare caseworkers, physical therapists, occupational therapists, clinical psychotherapists, and volunteers.
- Health care at home program during the third year of the medical curricula. This is a mandatory subject (one credit) where students are sent to visiting nurse stations in Tokyo for 1 week and visit homes with district nurses. Nurses teach medical students.
- Working at a hospital during the fourth year of the medical curricula. This is a mandatory subject (one credit) where students are sent to the nursing department in the ward, the dietary department, and the pharmacy for 1 week. Students learn their respective roles through participating in multidisciplinary endeavors.
- Workshop for patient safety. The workshop is organized on the third Saturday of every month at 13:00–17:00, when a wide range of university and hospital staff members attend and participate in group discussions on patient safety. The group consists of a fifth-year medical student, a nursing student, a clinical technician, an office employee, a doctor, a resident, and two nurses (eight persons). The workshop helps students appreciate how office employees and technicians care for patients. This workshop became a mandatory subject in the fifth-year medical curricula in FY2004 and for nursing students in FY2005. This subject also provides an excellent opportunity for students to collaborate with a variety of health professionals in the hospital.

Medical students from the first year to the fifth year are expected to learn the following through the above-mentioned programs.

- Learn on the job. Passive learning is not suitable for acquiring the ability to appreciate multidisciplinary work. We considered it appropriate to learn through active and practical experience, particularly in on-the-job training. We chose the method where students must go to the workplace for 1 week, take responsibility for even small things, and work together with leaders.
- Develop the capacity to reflect on oneself. IPE is conducted on the job; hence, students are expected to follow rules in the workplace and to discipline themselves as others do. This is to "behave like a Roman when in Rome." It is required here to think of how to behave by observing the norms as well as to reflect on how one's behavior is seen in other people's eyes. Observing norms, reflecting on oneself, and improving one's behavior is called "reflective practice." We intend

to provide an educational environment where students reflect on themselves so they act in a way that other people think is correct and proper and eventually attain the ability to work in teams.
- Multidisciplinary collaboration. Collaboration across disciplines is of utmost importance nowadays in health care and other professional fields. The IPE program is a tool to nourish multidisciplinary collaboration. A single professional can no longer complete a task by him- or herself nowadays. It is necessary for a professional to collaborate with other professionals in teams to produce an outcome. Undergraduate professional education must build such collaborative capability.

3 Multidisciplinary Health Professions Education Programs

1. Community service for the handicapped program during the first year of the medical curriculum (mandatory subject, one credit).
2. Care for severely handicapped children and incurable patietns program during the second year (elective subject, one credit), two to five students per year. The Care for Severely Handicapped Children program and Support for Child Rearing in the Community program have been mandatory subjects since FY2009 (one credit each).
3. Health care at home during the third year (mandatory subject, one credit).
4. Working at a hospital during the fourth year (mandatory, one credit).
5. Workshop for patient safety during the fifth year (mandatory, 4 hours). (This workshop was renamed the "Workshop for Teamwork Building at a Hospital" in FY2009.)

4 Organizational Structure of the Programs

The IPE program of the Jikei University began in FY1989 as the medical subject entitled, "Nursing Care Practice for Medical Students." This subject was made possible by the strong leadership of then President Masakazu Abe. The Educational Committee (the highest executive structure of faculty education) managed the program. The University introduced the systematic working experience training program in 1996 during extensive revision of the curriculum of the Department of Medicine. The revision, led by former President Tetsuo Okamura, was proposed and implemented after a thorough review of the whole school's education programs. Under the current President Satoshi Kurihara, the program has been expanded. Now, the program will have new inclusions with programs called "Care for Severely Handicapped Children" (working experience training at rehabilitation and nursery centers and schools for disabled children in Tokyo) and "Support for Child Rearing in the Community" (children's halls, nursery schools, and child-rearing support projects in Tokyo).

As mentioned above, the IPE program at the Jikei University School of Medicine was introduced under the leadership of the presidents for three generations as a result of extensive reviews of the whole school's education programs. Currently, the IPE program of the Department of Medicine was implemented with the Introduction to General Medicine under the supervision of the Educational Committee. It includes various professionals who teach students IPE at their working places, instead of the students learning it from the academic staff of the university. An educational workshop is organized to prepare a trainer staff who supervise health care at home during the third year of the medical curriculum (once a year on a Saturday from 10:00 to 16:00) At the workshop, lectures are provided on education theories, outcome evaluation, and feedback skills; in addition, discussions take place on how to assist students. Other efforts are made regarding health care at home, in addition to the workshop mentioned above. The member of the staff in charge of the program (a professor at the Center for Medical Education) visits the training sites of the 35 visiting nurse stations after the student practice and asks for information and opinions about student's attitudes and behavior and then performs student evaluation. At the same time, the professor studies the teaching methodology used and the feedback done for the students at each station. The study results are shared with each station at the time of the next visit, contributing to sharing the experience in the stations.

5 Outcomes of the Programs

The programs, through clinical training at a hospital during upper school years, aim at preparing students to work collaboratively in teams with diverse professionals, serve communities with improved care, and learn from patients. It is currently difficult to evaluate educational outcomes directly. However, it is possible to evaluate outcomes, to some extent, using evaluations by graduates of the medical school who were the primary stakeholders in the program.

In 2006, a questionnaire survey for graduates was conducted, with the findings indicated below.

1. Are you satisfied with the whole medical education program?—highly satisfactory 9.9%, satisfactory 80.3% (positive in 90.2%)
2. What do you think of the "social welfare training program"? very good 42.3%, good 49.3% (positive 91.6%)
3. What do you think of the "care-at-home program"? Very good 38.0%, good 52.1% (positive 90.1%)
4. What do you think of the "hospital practice training program"? very good 21.1%, good 46.5% (positive 67.6%)
5. Example comment: "It was excellent to get practice experience from lower school years in medicine, health, and welfare under training programs such as social welfare or care at home. This enabled me to become sensitive to view-

points of patients and service users. Currently, I am working at a general hospital. I understand that graduates from other universities have not had such experiences, and hence I sometimes feel that their views are narrow."

Obviously, graduates highly valued the programs.

A report of a fifth-year student gave the following evaluation of the patient safety workshop.

> I have been going through clinical training for about 1 year now. I think that this workshop was a good opportunity for me to on reflect clinical training. I realize that a big difference exists between previous classroom studies and clinical training. I mean that it is textbooks I learn from under the former but patients under the latter. Clinical training is not a place for me to study but a place for solving patient problems. It is not that patients come to hospital to help my study. Hence, although we are still students, we have to think of serving patients and have to study health care, skills, and knowledge as a means for it. Such an attitude must be maintained throughout a professional career, let alone at university.

Part of another report by a fourth-year medical student who received training at the rehabilitation hospital for 4 days under an elective subject stated the following.

> I learned the importance of team-based medicine, but I have had doubts about it in actual clinical settings. The hospital where I received training has established a collaborative system where various professions serve patients in teams. I realized that the hospital is not a teaching hospital because it did not "teach" me. Under previous training, I expected to be taught as a matter of course. However, nobody at the hospital had spare time to teach me. Being left alone, I was doing nothing initially and regretted that I had chosen the hospital as a training site. But later I approached patients and staff on my own, raised questions, touched patients' hands gently, and chatted. I found such experiences enjoyable and useful. I came to realize that I had lived in an environment where I was cared for but there was no active effort or participation on my part. This time, I assisted both doctors and co-medicals, and hence I obtained both viewpoints. Afresh, I felt glad when patients recovered.

These comments indicate that the programs encourage students to grow as professionals and human beings.

6 Overall Features of the Program

There is evidence that students improve their attitude and behavior when interprofessional collaboration training is conducted systematically every school year. Roughly 10 to 20 first-year students prove problematic each year according to the findings of interviews at training facilities after social welfare training. Those students received feedback about their behavior and, if necessary, receive instructions from their teachers face to face. However, problematic students decreased to two or three when the same group of students entered the third school year, according to an evaluation of care at home training. It is suggested that the feedback during the first school year urged students to reflect on themselves and change their behavior. The evaluation results of the third school year care at home training are fed back to all students and encourage further self-reflection.

It is also expected that the program should cultivate students' capacity to learn at the workplace. A student commented after the training that the goal of the clinical training was to contribute to patients. Thus, even students recognize that learning is a process of expanding their areas of responsibility, starting from small ones.

Various hospital professionals commented that they were reminded of what they had forgotten after joining the workforce thanks to group discussions with students at the patient safety workshop. This clearly indicates an aspect of IPE where students themselves are a source of education for other professionals. In fact, under IPE programs students not only learn from various professionals, they often educate them.

Interprofessional Education at the Keio University Faculty of Pharmacy

Yoshihiro Ehara, Yoshihiro Abe, Kazuko Fujimoto, Noriko Fukushima, Shiro Iijima, Satoko Ishikawa, Keiko Kishimoto, Mayumi Mochizuki, Kyoko Takahashi, Eriko Yokota, and Shizuko Kobayashi

Summary

As part of a trial course on interprofessional education (IPE) at Keio University our Faculty of Pharmacy initiated a joint seminar with the university's medical and nursing departments in 2008. We had two joint seminars: one in June and another in October. In the seminars, students and participants actively discussed several issues with regard to the national and private health care systems and medical malpractice. They also listened to feedback lectures held by experts from the medical and social system. At Kyoritsu University of Pharmacy, we had already held similar joint seminars three times since 2006. The participants were not only from our school but from various universities around Japan, given that our school was then only a small college for pharmaceutical students. Our considerable experience in the field of small group learning (SGL) helped make these seminars a success. By making full use of the SGL method we have successfully lead the discussion sessions at the IPE seminars attended by students from various medical fields. After the merging of our small pharmaceutical college with Keio University, we continued holding joint seminars for the three medical faculties at Keio University. It has not been without tribulations, however. The newly created interprofessional seminars faced several problems. The seeming lack of interest

---

Faculty of Pharmacy, Keio University, 1-5-30 Shibakohen, Minato-ku, Tokyo 105-8512, Japan
Tel. +81-3-3434-6241; Fax +81-3-3434-5343
e-mail: ehara-ys@pha.keio.ac.jp

Correspondence to: Y. Ehara

The authors are members of the SGL Committee 2006–2008

shown by the medical school decreased the level of participation of medical students, while too many facilitators are required for such seminars. To resolve these issues, we have made some changes to future activities in this area. To start with, we plan to change the course from an elective to a required subject for the students of the three medical faculties in Keio University.

Key words Interprofessional education · Joint seminars · Small group learning· Merging · Tribulations

1 Background

Keio University Faculty of Pharmacy is a new faculty that was founded in April 2008. Interprofessional education (IPE), however, already started with a joint seminar for students from several university medical faculties held at the former Kyoritsu University of Pharmacy in November 2006. It was one of the projects supported by the Ministry of Education, Culture, Sports, Science, and Technology, Japan, for "training high-quality medical professionals," and mainly a tutorial group learning for undergraduates supervised by the Small Group Learning (SGL) Committee established in 2003. The committee made use of the SGL method. The classes were at first an extracurricular activity conducted with the aid of several voluntary assistants, in which about 30 undergraduates took part and discussed medical problems such as diseases or medical malpractice in small groups. From these experiences, the committee recognized how necessary it was for the tutors (or facilitators) to be trained and to hold tutors' workshops. In 2005, the committee switched the extracurricular class to a regular, but elective, class, and put it into practice, although it was only for pharmaceutical students.

The turning point came in 2006. That year a new system for pharmacy education in Japan began and required that pharmaceutical students study 6 years before becoming pharmacists. One of its purposes was to enable students to acquire training in ethics and humanity as well as in solving problems. To meet this requirement we changed the course in bioethics (a required subject) from a lecture-style to a group-style learning to encourage the students to raise issues and then solve them. Moreover, we added two subjects to the curriculum—presentation skills and information technology—and have constructed a course made up of three subjects titled "To appreciate the value of life."

For as many as 180 students to take part in the program, there were two difficulties to overcome. For one thing, we had to prepare a large space that could be divided into two: one for lectures and one for group workshops. For another, we needed many facilitators to take care of the 13–15 groups per school hour. It was funds, however, that were most necessary to manage the course. As a result, we applied for financial aid to "the promotion program of the Ministry of Education, Culture, Sports, Science, and Technology–Japan for training high quality medical professionals." We were successful. The proposal to the ministry depicted a joint seminar for students from several medical faculties—e.g., medicine, pharmacy, nursing—from different universities, where the students would come together and discuss matters concerning medicine and health care.

In 2005, it was indispensible for Kyoritsu University of Pharmacy (which at that time was only a small college of pharmacy) to form a consortium with the nearest medical colleges to study and discuss regional medical services. Fortunately, some colleges—medical schools and a school of nursing—accepted our offer; and a joint seminar for students not only from these colleges but from others all over Japan was realized. In 3 years (2006–2008), we have had three seminars, where students of different medical fields eagerly discussed a range of subjects.

The seminars were a great success because we had already become experienced in the SGL method, and the space and facilities for it were well equipped. It was in this way that IPE was initiated into the Keio University Faculty of Pharmacy. During 2008, at the time of this writing, we have already had two seminars with students from three faculties—medicine, pharmacy, nursing—at Keio University.

2 Joint Seminars 2007–2008

Joint seminar 1

Date and time: March 22, 2007; 10:00–17:20
Place: Memorial Hall, Kyoritsu University of Pharmacy
Theme: Malpractice

Case 1: Anticancer drug overdose
Case 2: Decision-making by ovarian cancer patient

Feedback lecture: Teamwork in the ward (in the case of Nutrition Support Team)

Joint seminar 2

Date and time: August 10, 2007; 10:00–18:00
Place: Memorial Hall, Kyoritsu University of Pharmacy
Theme: Terminal care and palliative care—learning from cancer patients/the terminal care front (based on a TV program)
Feedback lectures: Psychological support in palliative care/Nursing in the face of death/The role of pharmacists in palliative care

Joint seminar 3

Date and time: August 8, 2008; 10:00–17:30
Place: Memorial Hall, Keio University Faculty of Pharmacy
Theme: Home care in the future—improving the quality of life of both patients and families

Case 1: Dementia
Case 2: Cerebral infarction
Case 3: Cancer

Panel discussion: The prospects of home care in the future by doctor, nurse, pharmacist, and occupational/physical therapist (OT/PT)

The process is the same for all seminars, and the aim is to encourage students to generate many opinions on a theme by examining it from various aspects.

The students are divided into 13–15 groups. Each group is required to discuss the chosen case and present a result. They need to work intensively and within a limited time. Some students were not satisfied because the time was too short to consider matters in depth, although they found some fulfillment in their intensive work. In any case, it was certain that the participants had a productive time, and the first aim of students from different medical faculties understanding each other was achieved. We can also guess this from the participants' positive responses in their evaluation forms.

Next, it was time to present their results to all the other participants. The groups make presentations in various ways. In some groups, one person is chosen, whereas in others all members explain in turn. In any case, we can see from the presentations how thoroughly the groups have discussed their subject.

Finally, there are feedback lectures by experts concerning the theme, and/or there are medical staff members who comment and offer presentations on their special knowledge and experience. The first and second seminars were held in this style; while in the third seminar, panel discussions were adopted so the students could listen to various panelists. Scenes from the seminars are shown in Figs. 1–4.

3 Percentage of Students from Each Faculty

The number and percentage of participants in these three joint seminars (JS), with regard to faculty, are as follows.

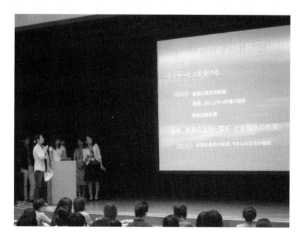

Fig. 1. A scene of presentation

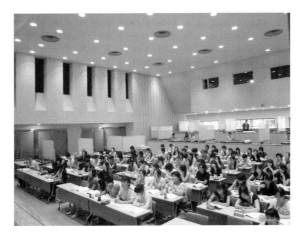

Fig. 2. Listening to a feedback lecture

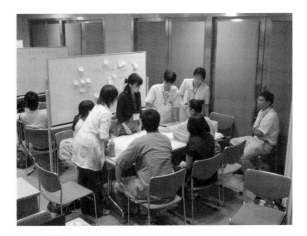

Fig. 3. Participation in a group workshop

JS 1: 100 students; nursing 28%, pharmacy 30%, medicine 15%, others 27%
JS 2: 118 students; nursing 42%, pharmacy 29%, medicine 16%, others 13%
JS 3: 105 students; nursing 44%, pharmacy 39%, medicine 7%, others 10%

4 Student Evaluations (from Questionnaire Results)

The aim of the seminars was to create an environment where the participants from various medical professions, while still students, can deepen their understanding of

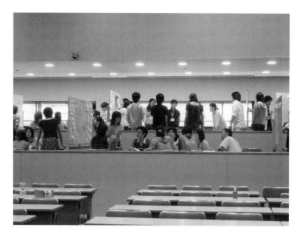

Fig. 4. Watching a presentation

Table 1. Questionnaire results, based on a scale of 1–5

Questions		JS 1	JS 2	JS 3
No. of participants		100	118	105
Q1.	Did you find any difficulty coming to today's workshop?	4.2	3.9	4.1
Q2.	Do you think that this seminar will be useful for you in the future?	4.7	4.5	4.6
Q3.	Did you discuss well?	4.3	4.1	4.2
Q4.	Did today's theme meet your requirements?	4.4	4.1	4.3

JS, joint seminar

each other and express their opinions openly and without fear. The most important evaluation was how willingly they participated and actively discussed the subject at hand because many of them met for the first time.

Questionnaire results are shown in Table 1. It is satisfying to note that we obtained a very high score on the second question in Table 1. However, we also have concerns about the medical systems of the future—whether they will measure up to students' expectations.

The answers most commonly given by the participants to two questions are as follows.

Q1. What did you mainly learn from the seminar?

- It is valuable to exchange opinions during our student days with those who will go into various medical fields.
- I have understood the ways of thinking of students from other faculties.
- The importance of medical treatment coordinated by a team consisting of doctors, nurses, pharmacists, and other medical staffs.
- The importance of communication among medical staff.
- The place my own profession occupies among other professions.

Q2. What is not enough? What should be improved?

- We should have more time for discussion to deepen our own point of view.
- It might be better to have more time for discussions than for presentations.
- There were too few participants from medical schools and faculties of social welfare.

From these answers, we recognized that too few medical students participated in the seminar and it was the greatest problem. Furthermore, most students understood the importance of interprofessional workshops and of patient care developed by teams from various medical professions.

5 Future Problems and Prospects

The two seminars in 2007 were interesting and useful not only for the students from Kyoritsu University of Pharmacy but also for us, the members of the SGL Committee. Pharmaceutical students, during the short period of 4 years, had far less actual experience than students from medical and nursing faculties. It was therefore stimulating and encouraging to discuss and learn together with the medical students, and at times it seemed as if we had made contact with a foreign culture.

It was decided that our college should be absorbed into Keio University and become one of the medical faculties of the university just when we were going to put the idea of a joint curriculum into practice. It was certain at that point that IPE would be far easier to realize. In 2008, as of this writing, we have already held two seminars at Keio University. However, certain problems remain: (1) The three medical faculties of Keio University are physically far from each other; (2) there are too few participants from the medical school at the seminars; and (3) most of the teaching staff have little interest in such seminars.

There are, nevertheless, some good prospects. It will be possible to change the seminar from an elective to a required subject by having it be common to all the schools—it is key to have the medical students actively take part. From now on, the seminars will be held at the three medical faculties of Keio University, and other medical universities will join in. However, these seminars will not become a required subject in the near future.

Support Program for Contemporary Educational Needs: "Contemporary Good Practice" Project at Chiba University

Educational Program for Training Autonomous Health Care Professionals: Human Resource Training Emphasizing Interprofessional Collaboration

Misako Miyazaki[1], Ikuko Sakai[1], Tomoko Majima[1], Itsko Ishii[2], Yuko Sekine[2], Masahiro Tanabe[3], Mayumi Asahina[3], Hotaka Noguchi[3], Narumi Ide[1], and Kieko Iida[1] (Chiba University Inohana IPE Working Group)

Summary

Medical care is an organized service made possible by the cooperation of numerous professionals. With the bachelor's degree as a basis of career education, education which students can gain not only technical knowledge but also enable them to show their professionalism based on the concept "patient (user)-centered care" as a member of a medical organization is vital. Above all, it is essential fostering students' abilities to work inter-professionally which might become a driving force of a team medical care. The present project covers all students in all grades from the Departments of Nursing, Medicine, and Pharmacy; and it provides multistage and comprehensive interprofessional education through lectures, drills, and practical training. The core of the program is the fostering of communication skills, ethical sensitivity, and problem-solving skills. This program is designed to train autonomous health care professionals with healthy occupational views, a strong sense of social responsibility, a sound work ethic, well-balanced views, and a willingness to commit to lifelong learning.

---

[1]School of Nursing, Graduate School of Nursing, Chiba University, 1-8-1 Inohara, Chuo-ku, Chiba 260-8672, Japan
Tel. +81-43-226-2435; Fax +81-43-226-2435
e-mail: miyamisa@faculty.chiba-u.jp
[2]Faculty of Pharmaceutical Sciences, Graduate School of Pharmaceutical Sciences, Chiba University, Chiba, Japan
[3]School of Medicine, Graduate School of Medicine, Chiba University, Chiba, Japan

Correspondence to: M. Miyazaki

Key words Undergraduated compulsory multistage program · Health care professionals · Communication skills · Ethical sensitivity · Problem-solving skills

1 Profile and Mission of Chiba University

At Chiba University, the three health care departments—medicine, pharmacy, and nursing—are located on the Inohana campus. Chiba University is the only national administrative institution with three academic departments that have long histories and rich traditions. In the past, independent educational systems pursued highly specialized fields of study. Although instructors from the Department of Medicine have given lectures on pathology and therapy in the Department of Nursing and the Department of Pharmacy, there have been few opportunities for all three departments to participate equally in basic education.

Chiba University is a core of highly advanced medical care and regional alliances, which are necessary for the high-quality medicine that modern society demands. It is expected to educate members of the medical community who can provide high-quality care. At Chiba University, a project has been initiated to promote a program that constitutes an advanced trial in cooperation among the three clinical schools with good partnerships.

2 Background and Goals of the IPE Program

We believe that health care professionals who can independently promote team medicine are needed for better health care. Hence, with a discretionary budget prepared by the Director of the Nursing Department in 2005 and by the President in 2006, our working group visited an English university to study interprofessional education (IPE). By then reviewing cases in Japan and the relevant literature, the Inohana Interprofessional Education Program (Inohana IPE) was developed to facilitate interprofessional collaboration among the three health care departments at Chiba University. The program was implemented in 2007.

2.1 Goals of the Project

Inohana IPE is designed for students in health care departments—nursing, medicine, pharmacy—to develop their professional identity through patient (user)-centered medicine and to acquire the basic skills for continuously developing their careers as health care professionals. The program emphasizes interprofessional collaboration, which is at the core of patient-centered medicine. Educational courses are developed and verified to further improve and advance education methods.

2.2 Goals of IPE and Desired Human Resources

The three keys to successful patient-centered medicine are communication skills, ethical sensitivity, and problem-solving skills. Thus the educational goal of Inohana IPE is to help students acquire these skills. Through this type of educational approach, Inohana IPE is designed to train autonomous health care professionals with healthy occupational views, a strong sense of social responsibility, a sound work ethic, well-balanced views, and willingness to commit to lifelong learning.

2.3 Educational Content of the IPE Program

Inohana IPE is a multistage, long-term, systematic program that is designed to foster communication skills, medical ethics, and problem-solving skills to provide patient- or user-centered medicine. Inohana IPE is managed with equal collaboration and cooperation among the departments of nursing, medicine, and pharmacy.

Inohana IPE has four steps, and each step has defined learning goals as follows.

- Step 1—"Sharing." The aim of this step is to form the foundation for promoting team medicine by understanding patients and users, acquiring better communication skills, and respecting and valuing other health care professionals.
- Step 2—"Creation." This step helps the students understand team building, team management, and interprofessional collaboration. Also included is the aim to assist them in creating new interprofessional teams independently and improve patient-centered medicine before and after entry into practice. This also helps students develop broad views and flexible thinking so they can guide team medicine to new directions in the future.
- Step 3—"Solution." The aim of this step is to allow students to participate in decision-making, addressing ethical issues through interprofessional collaboration, and to acquire techniques for dealing with various problems while focusing on patients.
- Step 4—"Integration." The purpose of this step is to implement team medicine in clinical settings by integrating the knowledge and skills for interprofessional collaboration that are acquired throughout the first three steps. This stimulates networking and sharing of best educational approaches for collaborative patient-centered practice.

Nursing is a 4-year program, and medicine and pharmacy are 6-year programs. Figure 1 shows the completion schedule of each step in each department. Table 1 outlines the structure of the Inohana IPE program. Students must complete each step before moving on to the next. Steps 1 and 2 are completed before taking

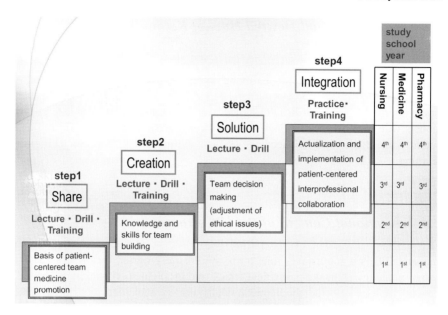

Fig. 1. Summary of the Inohana interprofessional education model

specialist subjects, and steps 3 and 4 are completed after students take certain specialist subjects.

2.4 Characteristics of the IPE program

2.4.1 IPE: Compulsory Subject Based on Mutual Respect for the Existing Curricula of the Three Schools

Inohana IPE is set up as a compulsory subject with the agreement of the three schools. It is essential for medical personnel training and for securing the quality of the University's medical care educational system for future doctors, nurses, and pharmacists.

2.4.2 Implementation System

Interprofessional education is the core of the present project, and its goal is to improve the quality of health care by encouraging professionals in various fields to collaborate with one another. IPE facilitates students/professionals in different departments studying together and understanding each other's roles through mutual learning. In this regard, IPE is different from multiprofessional education where

Table 1. Structure of Inohana IPE program

Structure	Learning goals	Learning contents	Location, methods, etc./class formats
Step 1 (sharing)	Acquire the necessary communication skills for promoting patient/user-centered team medicine	Understand patients (users) Learn the necessary basic communication skills for team medicine Professionals in the insurance, medicine, and welfare fields need to respect each other	Lectures and drills: campus Practical training: medical institutions such as the university hospital
Step 2 (creation)	Possess the necessary knowledge for effective team building by ascertaining the occupational role and function of each team member	Acquire the necessary basic knowledge for team building Acquire the necessary knowledge for team management Understand interprofessional teams in clinical settings and become aware of function and collaboration	Lectures and drills: campus Practical training: community care facilities, public health centers, medical facilities, nursing facilities
Step 3 (solution)	Have the common goal of patient-centered medicine and learn techniques to solve problems as a team	Understand the necessary communication skills to address and solve team conflicts Learn techniques for making decisions in interprofessional collaboration Learn techniques to address ethics in team settings	Lectures and drills: university Drills: review records of patient conferences (e.g., video), experience real team decision-making processes, and learn ethical sensitivity through hypothetical patients and case studies Lectures: medical ethics and techniques for solving ethical dilemmas
Step 4 (integration)	Learn about professional behaviors to achieve patient-centered interprofessional collaboration	Learn the practical techniques to design and implement patient care therapy through interprofessional collaboration	Lectures and drills: campus (meaning of IPE, attitude and behaviors as good health care professionals, self-assessment through portfolios) Practical training: university hospital, etc. (experience actual therapy; learn care plan designing and implementation with interprofessional collaboration through clinical training in each department)

professionals in different fields learn together irrespective of goals and objectives.

The present project covers all students in all grades from the Departments of Nursing, Medicine, and Pharmacy. It provides multistage, comprehensive interprofessional education through lectures, drills, and practical training. The core of the program is the fostering of communication skills, ethical sensitivity, and problem-solving skills. After each practical training session, there is time for students to review events and their feelings, thereby finding meaning that deepens their knowledge and their understanding of the process.

2.4.2.1 Management and Instructors

The Interprofessional Education Promotion Committee comprises instructors from the three departments (i.e., medicine pharmacy, nursing). The committee is responsible for project planning and design, coordination, adjustment, and assessment. The committee works with the "Instruction Office" of each department to choose instructors and teaching assistants (TAs).

A great deal of work is involved in developing, implementing, and verifying education assessment methods, faculty development, and staff development (see section 2.4.2.2). Therefore, one program coordinator (part-time, PhD) and one office assistant are assigned to promote and assist the Interprofessional Education Promotion Committee.

2.4.2.2 Support System

In terms of training facilities, in collaboration with the Chiba University Hospital, students learn in the Comprehensive Medical Education Training Center, the Department of Nursing, and the Department of Pharmacy.

Many instructors, TAs, and collaborators (health care professionals at training facilities) are involved, and it is important for these individuals to understand clearly the objective of the present program and improve leadership skills for interprofessional collaboration. Hence, the Interprofessional Collaboration Promotion Committee plans and implements faculty development and staff development.

2.4.2.3 Extramural Collaboration

- *Collaboration with medical institutions within the prefecture*: To expand the circle of training facilities beyond the university hospital, it is necessary to explore model areas for IPE and to collaborate with extramural medical institutions. This solidifies the implementation system of the program and develops the necessary skills for interprofessional collaboration.

- *Collaborating and networking with other schools*: It is necessary to communicate periodically, forming a network, with domestic and overseas universities that are also tackling IPE. This networking contributes to the development of the ethics and methodologies of IPE.

3 Efficacy of the IPE Program

An outline of the method used to evaluate the Inohana IPE is presented in Table 2.[1] We are thus developing an evaluation process by accumulating data by testing the efficacy, the processes, and the effects of the program.

In contrast, the students are judged by their teachers regarding their accomplishments based on their scholastic records and reports on the students. Unfortunately, scholastic evaluation bias is rampant because the teachers do not unify certain criteria among themselves. Therefore, a working group is discussing the educational effects and the methods of evaluating the educational process. For example, the working group members discuss whether student performance checks during the classes should be included on evaluation process not just assessed by their reports and self-evaluations, in order to evaluate students' changes in attitude and knowledge acquisition as results of IPE.

Table 2. Parameters and materials of evaluation

Parameter	Concrete contents	Points of evaluation
Outcome	Manner formation	A prior report
	Improvement of recognition	Final report of the student
	Acquisition of knowledge	Results of group work
	Acquisition of a skill	Group interview
	Change in behavior	
Process	Satisfaction and achievement of students	Reflection sheet
	Participation situation of students	Minutes paper
	Administration situation of students	Group interview
	Education methods	Class evaluation by the students
		Feedback by the teacher and TA
Effect	Influence on teachers	Questionnaire to the teacher and TA regarding cooperation, attendance, and response to faculty development
	Influence on training sites	Questionnaire to the training institution, IPW enforcement situation at the site, listening to the person in charge
	Influence on patients concerned	Listening to patients and persons concerned
	Influence on university	Listening to administration sections of the university and its hospital

TA, teacher's assistant; IPW, interprofessional work

4 Discussion

4.1 Promotion Factors for the Inohana IPE Project

To promote IPE strongly, it is important to plan specific IPE projects that include positive features of our own university in a way that complies with the educational philosophy of the university. In addition, it is important to attain feedback that is always conscious of the purposes of IPE—"Who is to benefit from IPE? What are the goals of IPE?"—from stakeholders who are the teachers, professionals in the field, and the administration of the university, among others. Because the strengths and weaknesses are different at each university, we cannot follow the route of an already developed program at another institution. We have to analyze our own organization from various angles, after which we should design a program that we are best able to plan practically on a realistic basis.

In the case of Inohana IPE, when there was a clash of opinions among teachers of the three schools, resulting in opposition and conflicts, we were able to continue talks, by always returning to our basic goals: to establish a patient/service user-centered program; to make the program a compulsory subject in all three schools; and to adopt a learning method that allows students to see the deep significance of their actions during learning experiences. It is important as well that teachers respect and learn from each other during this process. We did indeed complete the main project because we shared its aims and thus saved most of our energy to adjust to the ideas of the educational committees of the three schools. These committees, fortunately, had already recognized the need for educational reform and had reformed it in the past by curriculum revision. Therefore, it was easy to get cooperation for enforcement of the Inohana IPE program, and it was administered as scheduled.

4.2 Problems of Inohana IPE

A weak point of the Inohana IPE is that opportunities to work with faculties and students from the field of social work/service have not provided. This poses a risk that the program and students' learning become rather "medical care-centered". Our task at the present is to secure opportunities for students to learn and accept diversity of people's ways of thinking and values in the social context which cannot be separated from the medical care.

Although there are mutual understandings between the members of the working group for the most part, there are differences in values which are difficult to overcome, particularly between different schools. For instance, to reach consensus on how students support should be provided and on setting up the ideal standard of scholastic evaluation between the students and the faculties in the three schools is difficult. This cannot be done by simply sharing the methods because student support and evaluation are the two sides of the same coin. These two are the value system of the education, in other word, the educational "faith".

It is difficult to cultivate interprofessionalism in Inohana IPE—that is, an attitude of altruism, awareness of obligations and actions, and ethics—as it deeply depends on personal experiences and their meaning as well as pursuing one's own profession.[2]

Acknowledgments This work was supported in part by a grant from the Ministry of Education, Culture, Sports, Science, and Technology.

References

1. Miyazaki M, Sakai I, Ide N, et al (2008) The development of learning outcome evaluation items for interprofessional education in Japan. Presented at the Association for Medical Education in Europe 2008 Conference, p 129
2. Robinson M, Cottrell D (2005) Health professionals in multi-disciplinary and multi-agency teams: changing professional practice. J Interprof Care 19:547–560

Interprofessional Team-Based Medical Education Program at Kitasato University: Collaboration Among 14 Health-Related Professions

Kiyohisa Mizumoto[1], Makito Okamoto[2], Kunio Ishii[3], Makoto Noshiro[4], Yuko Kuroda[5], Masuo Shirataka[6], Masaki Taga[7], Kaoru Iguchi[8], Hisashi Ikemoto[9], and Tadayoshi Shiba[1]

Summary

Medical technology is quickly becoming more advanced and more narrowly specialized. At the same time, epidemiological and demographic profiles are changing drastically. Therefore, it would be difficult to provide the utmost health services unless various pieces of knowledge scattered across multiple health-related professions are integrated for practical application. Furthermore, as society's needs for health services are also changing, it is no longer enough to treat the disease. Hence, the quality of health services is being looked at to humanize the process of diagnosis and treatment and to consider ethical, psychological, and social aspects of services. To provide quality health services, it is imperative for various health-related professionals, who are narrowly specialized, to closely work together as a

---

[1] Kitasato University, 5-9-1 Shirokane, Minato-ku, Tokyo 108-8641, Japan
Tel. +81-3-3444-6161(ext. 3317); Fax +81-3-3442-5674
e-mail: mizumoto@kitasato-u.ac.jp
[2] School of Medicine, Kitasato University, Sagamihara, Kanagawa, Japan
[3] School of Pharmacy, Kitasato University, Shirokane, Minato, Tokyo, Japan
[4] School of Allied Health Sciences, Kitasato University, Sagamihara, Kanagawa, Japan
[5] School of Nursing, Kitasato University, Sagamihara, Kanagawa, Japan
[6] College of Liberal Arts and Sciences, Kitasato University, Sagamihara, Kanagawa, Japan
[7] Kitasato Junior College of Health and Hygienic Sciences, Minami-Uonuma, Niigata, Japan
[8] Kitasato Nursing School, Kitamoto, Saitama, Japan
[9] Education Center, Kitasato University, Sagamihara, Kanagawa, Japan

Correspondence to: K. Mizumoto

team. This, in turn, requires urgent training of human resources so that such collaborative teamwork can smoothly take place.

Kitasato University has four health-related schools and two specialized colleges, which together educate as many as 14 types of health-related specialist professionals. The university is also known for its good clinical education in collaboration with its four affiliated hospitals. By taking advantage of these unique characteristics, the university, as a whole, embarked on the Interprofessional Team-Based Medical Education Program in 2006 as one of its key educational programs. The Program, built on the conventional school education method (so-called "vertical education"), which had already proven effective, aims to train students through collaboration among different professionals with specifically innovated educational methods and contents to encourage such collaboration. Through this "cross-sectional education," students gain the ability to collaborate effectively with others.

Currently, the Program includes (1) the All-Kitasato Team-Based Medical Drill, which is a simulated team-based medical exercise undertaken by small groups consisting of 10 students each. The drill started in 2006 and trains about 1200 senior students from the four health-related schools and two specialized colleges each year; and (2) An Introduction to Team-Based Medicine lecture, which started in 2008 as an introductory course common to all four health-related schools. It is meant to make the collaboration in health care more systematic. The lecture is given to about 1000 freshman students each year to deepen their understanding and appreciation of team-based medicine at an early stage of their university education. It is a real-time, two-way, dialogue-style, online lecture. As subsequent steps to initiatives (1) and (2) above, the university further plans to establish (3) Team-Based Clinical Training, which will be a practical training program conducted primarily at the four university-affiliated hospitals; and (4) a system-wide University Clinical Education Center, which will coordinate clinical education collaboration and team-based clinical training among the four university-affiliated hospitals and the four health-related schools.

Key words 4 health-related schools and 2 colleges · 14 health-related professions · 4 university-affiliated hospitals · Team-Based Medical Drill · Team-Based Medicine Lecture · System-wide University Clinical Education Center

1 Profile of Kitasato University

Kitasato University teaches fundamental biological and health sciences and consists of seven schools—Medicine, Pharmacy, Nursing, Allied Health Sciences, Sciences, Veterinary Medicine, Marine Bioscience—the college of Liberal Arts and Sciences, and the colleges of Health and Hygienic Sciences and Nursing. The university was founded in 1962 as the 50th anniversary project of the Kitasato Institute, which was Japan's first private medical research institution established in 1914 by

Shibasaburou Kitasato. Dr. Kitasato laid a number of important foundations in preventive medicine, such as bacteriology and immunology, including the successful pure culture of tetanus bacilli (*Clostridium tetani*) and the subsequent discovery of anti-tetanus toxin. Since its establishment, the university has aimed to produce competent researchers, educators, and other professionals in the fields of bioscience and medicine for the benefit of the society. This has been done with Kitasato's founding four principles, to which he adhered his entire life: "Investigate with a pioneering spirit." "Be appreciative in your dealings with people." "Possess wisdom and be a person of practical science." "Persist with an unwavering spirit."

The university has a School of Medicine (Faculty of Medicine); School of Pharmacy (Faculty of Pharmacy, a 6-year course) and Department of Pharmaceutical Sciences (4-year course); School of Nursing (Department of Nursing); and School of Allied Heath Sciences (Department of Health Sciences, Department of Medical Laboratory Sciences, Department of Medical Engineering and Technology, and Department of Rehabilitation). Each school has a postgraduate master's degree and doctorate courses. A separate postgraduate school, called the Graduate School of Medical Sciences, was set up for Schools of Medicine and Allied Health Sciences. As is explained later in this chapter, the university is known for its good clinical education realized through close collaboration with its four affiliated hospitals.

2 Background and Goals of Team-Based Medical Education Program

To provide patient-centered, high-quality, safe health services, it is imperative for a number of narrowly specialized health-related professionals to work closely together (i.e., team-based medicine). This, in turn, requires urgent training of human resources to be capable of such collaborative team work. Unfortunately, medical education so far in Japan has not addressed this urgent need enough.

Kitasato University has four health-related schools (i.e., Schools of Medicine, Pharmacy, Nursing, and Allied Health Sciences) and two colleges (i.e., Junior College of Health and Hygienic Sciences and the Nursing School). It trains its students to be proficient in 14 health-related professions (i.e., as physicians, pharmacists, nurses, midwives, public nurses, clinical laboratory technicians, clinical engineering technologists, radiology technologists, physical therapists, occupational therapists, speech-language-hearing therapists, orthoptists, health supervisors, and registered dietitians), all of which professions require national certification. The university is also known for its clinical education in close collaboration with its four affiliated hospitals: Kitasato University Hospital, Kitasato University East Hospital, Kitasato Institute Hospital, Kitasato Institute Medical Center (KMC) Hospital (Fig. 1). All four affiliated hospitals share common guiding principles of patient-centered medicine and collaborative medicine. The understanding that "Medicine is always a team-based exercise" prevails among people working there.

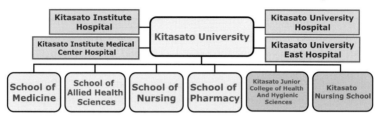

Fig. 1. Features of health-related education conducted by four health-related schools and two colleges of Kitasato University

Under this favorable environment, the university's Board of Directors decided to initiate the Interprofessional Team-Based Medical Education Program starting in 2006 as one of its key educational programs. Furthermore, the All Kitasato Team Medicine Drill was embarked on under the leadership of the University's Vice President and spearheaded by its Team Medicine Education Committee.

Recently, team-based medical education or interprofessional medical education have been advocated and initiated at some other medical educational institutions, including medical universities. However, the number of professions involved in such attempts varies. Under the favorable environment explained above, Kitasato University is well positioned to carry out interprofessional collaborative (team-based) medical education. By pursuing the Interprofessional Team-Based Medical Education Program, which involves as many as 14 professions, it is expected that the university can provide a distinctive model to this approach.

The objectives of this program are to help students in health-related schools (1) better understand the knowledge, skills, and expertise of other professions; (2) acquire the capacity to liaise and collaborate with other professions through mutual understanding and respect; and (3) acquire the capacity to serve patients holistically. To this end, the university has prepared educational programs and methodologies that are easy to understand and undertake as well as good for nurturing fundamental practical skills.

However, to go through team-based medical exercises effectively, each student must first learn the professional basics of his or her own school sufficiently to the extent that he or she has already established some professional identity. Therefore,

> **【General Instructional Objectives】**
> With the goal to take an active part in team-based medicine built on their own professions, to be able to address various medical and health care issues, and to provide patient-centered, high-quality medical services, students are expected to obtain basic knowledge, skills, and attitude about team-based medicine, a flow of medical services, and roles and responsibilities of health professions that form a medical team.
>
> **【Specific Behavioral Objectives】**
> ① To be able to list and explain health professions that are involved in team-based medical services
> ② To be able to clarify dependent and independent roles and responsibilities of each health professional
> ③ To be able to identify problems and issues of each health professional in case scenarios given and to be able to propose what could and should have been done on their side to amend situations
> ④ To be able to explain the meaning and goals of team-based medicine
> ⑤ To be able to clarify roles of patients in team-based medicine
> ⑥ To be able to plan health services from the view point of team-based medicine
> ⑦ To be able to communicate with other team members effectively

Fig. 2. General instructional objectives (GIO) and specific behavioral objectives (SBO) of team-based medicine education program at Kitasato University

it is also important to strengthen the students' conventional education ("vertical education") in each school. The concept of a System-wide University Clinical Education Center, explained later in the chapter, is expected to play a pivotal role in enriching not only the "lateral education"—cross-cutting school boundaries—but also the vertical/specialized education, in particular its clinical education/internship.

Figure 2 shows the general instructional objectives (GIOs) and specific behavioral objectives (SBOs) of the university's team medicine education. As is explained later, the SBOs are used as evaluation indicators.

3 Implementation Details of the Team-Based Medical Education Program

3.1 Team-based Medical Education Program's Priority in the University

As explained above, because Kitasato University has four health-related schools, two colleges, and four affiliated hospitals, it is well positioned to carry out the team-based medical education program. For example, unique educational programs involving many schools and professions, which would be rather difficult for other medical educational institutions to put together, could be structured at the university. Needless to say, however, each school already has its own tight curriculum, which varies in length from 3 to 6 years. Furthermore, geographically, the Schools of Medicine, Nursing, and Allied Health Sciences are located on the university's Sagamihara Campus in Kanagawa Prefecture, whereas the School of Pharmacy is located on its Shirokane Campus in Minato Ward of Tokyo, the College of Health and Hygienic Sciences on its Minami-Uonuma Campus in Niigata Prefecture, and its Nursing School on its Kitamoto Campus in Saitama Prefecture. Thus, it would be difficult to design curricula that necessitate students' logistical movements over a long period of time or, more so, involve students in their years of advanced studies. Therefore, initially, "An Introduction to the Team-Based Medicine," which was a common introductory lecture course for freshmen students of all schools, and the All-Kitasato Team-Based Medical Drill, which was meant for students in their advanced years, were introduced. Figure 3 shows the concepts of specialized education ("vertical education") and team-based

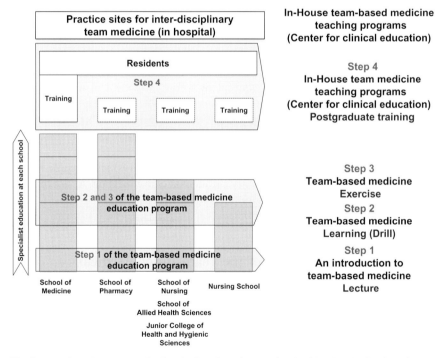

Fig. 3. Relations between professional education of respective health-related schools and team-based medical education. Steps 1 and 2 are ongoing, and step 3 is in the planning stage. Please refer to Fig. 7 for in-house clinical education centers

medical education program ("lateral education") schematically. Note that the current program does not necessarily correspond with the curriculum of each school for the number of school years.

The Introduction to Team-Based Medicine lecture is represented as step 1 in Fig. 3 and is meant for the first-year students of the Schools of Pharmacy, Nursing, and Allied Health Sciences and the third-year students of the School of Medicine (owing to constraints in its curriculum). This is a logical arrangement because all students of these schools start their general education courses at the university's Sagamihara Campus. The lecture course started in school year (SY) 2008 and is mandatory for students in the Schools of Medicine, Pharmacy, and Allied Health Sciences. (In SY2008, it became an optional course for the students of School of Nursing owing to the constraints of its curriculum.) Students in the two other colleges audit the lecture online. (School credits cannot be given to college students for taking online lectures.) As many as 12 classes were organized in the last semester.

The All-Kitasato Team-Based Medical Drill, represented as step 2 in Fig. 3, started in 2006. Third- or fourth-year students of the Schools of Pharmacy, Nursing, and Allied Health Sciences and fifth-year students of the School of Medicine participate in this drill, which is meant for students who have established some professional identities through their respective specialized courses. Each year, the drill is conducted during a full-2-day period in early May at the university's Sagamihara Campus, which is indeed an extra-large event attended by about 1200 students and 150 academic staff. About 1200 students are divided into 120 ten-member teams, each consisting of students from different schools, to have discussions and subsequent presentations based on simulated scenario cases. As is explained later, even though no credits are given for the drill, the participation rate of students has been very high.

3.2 All-Kitasato Team-Based Medical Drill in Pursuit of the Realization of Safer and Higher-Quality Health Services

To address various medical and health care issues and to provide patient-centered, high-quality medical services, about 1200 students from the Schools of Medicine (fifth year), Pharmacy (fourth year), Nursing (fourth year), Allied Health Sciences (third or fourth year), College of Health and Hygienic Sciences (third year or fourth year), and College of Nursing (third year) are invited to participate in the All-Kitasato Team-Based Medical Drill for 2 days. Participants form 10-member teams, each consisting of students from different schools (a total of 120 teams), discuss nine hypothetical assignments (simulated scenario/cases) (Table 1) in various health fields, and present the outcome of the discussion (e.g., it could be about the ideal team-based medical approach). The timetable of the 2-day event is shown in Table 2.

Table 1. Themes of the All-Kitasato Team-based Medical Drill (SY2008)

Theme no.	Theme	Subthemes
1	Emergency medicine	Acute treatment and cardiac rehabilitation of a myocardial infarction patient
2	Disaster medicine	Initial emergency medical response to a disaster
3	Infection control	Hospital infection control
4	Geriatric medicine	Home care of an elderly patient with dementia
5	Cerebrovascular medicine	Dysphagia, movement disorders, other complications of stroke
6	Pediatric oncology	Holistic support for a child suffering from advanced cancer
7	Diabetes mellitus (DM) medical management	DM and its complications
8	Neurological incurable disease management	Management of neurological incurable diseases
9	Lifestyle-related disease management	Variety of diseases occurring from unhealthy lifestyle patterns

Each team, consisting of 10 students from different schools, is given one of the nine themes. The team then discusses it over 2 days and reports the discussion's outcome. Scenarios are designed in such a way as to involve as many professions as possible

The discussion basically follows the KJ method, but its practical format is left for each team to decide. Discussion points are handwritten on four pages of flip charts, which are photographed by a digital camera, loaded into a personal computer (PC), and then processed into MS PowerPoint slides for presentation (Figs. 4, 5).

The necessary stationery, flip charts, notebook PC, and a digital camera are rented for each of the 120 teams. Small conference rooms for the exercise are temporarily equipped with a local area network (LAN) so all 120 teams can access the Internet. One facilitator (academic staff) assists each team. Facilitators evaluate the presentations, and good ones receive awards. The venue of the exercise is the university's Sagamihara Campus, and it is usually held over 2 days in early May. Three exercises have been held since 2006. The 2009 exercise (the fourth) was scheduled for May 1st and 2nd. Table 3 shows the number and percentage of students who participated in the exercise in 2008 by school/college. Of the total students, 86.3% participated in 2006, 94.2% in 2007, and 93.0% in 2008, which are considered quite high.

A questionnaire survey is carried out after the exercise that includes the students and the academic staff who participated in it. It is to find out the students' evaluation of the exercise (i.e., level of their satisfaction), the students' self-evaluation with respect to the SBOs, and the academic staff's evaluation of the students' achievement of the intended objectives. About 90% of the students

Table 2. Timetable of the "All-Kitasato Team-based Medical Drill"

Time	Agenda	Venue
First day		
9:00–9:20	Registration (confirmation of attendance)	Entrance of the main school building (Bldg. L3)
9:20–9:40	Welcome reception by the Chairperson of the Steering Committee (Vice President), Hospital Director, Faculty Directors	Middle-sized classrooms (each 130 seats) Large classroom (350 seats) Synchronous TV broadcasting
9:40–10:25	Opening session for briefing objectives, topics, method, and schedule by the Vice-Chairperson of the Steering committee	As above
10:25–10:40	Division into small teams	
10:40–11:00	Kickoff session for team discussion to introduce facilitators and members; have an icebreaker; designate roles to members	Small classrooms at each school building
11:00–12:10	Team discussions	As above
12:10–13:40	Lunch break	
13:40–15:40	Continuation of the team discussion	As above
15:40–15:55	Short break	
15:55–17:30	Continuation of the team discussion	
Second day		
9:00–9:20	Second-day orientation	Middle-sized classrooms (each 130 seats)
9:20–9:35	Division into small teams	
9:35–11:40	Continuation of the team discussion, wrap-up discussion, and preparation of the report	Small classrooms at each school building
11:40–13:10	Lunch break	
13:10–14:35	Plenary reporting session (first half—involves seven teams, 12 minutes each)	Bldg. L3—middle-sized classroom
14:35–14:50	Short break	
14:50–16:15	Plenary reporting session (latter half—involves seven teams, 12 minutes each); filling out questionnaires	As above
16:15–16:40	Transfer to the reception area	
16:40–18:00	Closing ceremony and farewell party for all participating students	Kitasato University gymnasium

responded "satisfied" or "slightly satisfied" with the exercise, and about 85% of them noted that they achieved the seven-item SBOs. The results indicated that most students who participated in the exercise properly understood its objectives, earnestly involved themselves in the assignment given, and acquired the intended skills. In this regard, it was found to be a big success. To further the academic staff's and students' appreciation of team-based medicine and its education, a "team-based medicine forum" is held at each campus (i.e., Shirokane Campus, Sagamihara Campus, Niigata Campus, and Saitama Campus) every year.

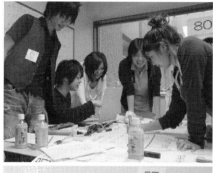
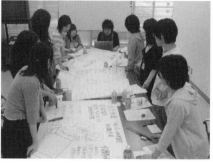
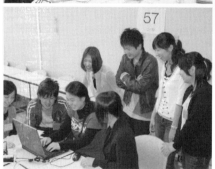

Fig. 4. All-Kitasato Team-Based Medical Drill for school year (SY)2008 (scene 1). A notebook personal computer is rented for each 10-member team (120 teams in all). Discussions take place on one of themes 1–9 (see Table 1)

3.3 Introduction to Team-Based Medicine: Common Introductory Course for All Health-Related Schools

The lecture course entitled Introduction to Team-Based Medicine aims to deepen the students' understanding of it at an early stage of their university education. The lecture provides fundamental knowledge required for team-based medicine, including the health care system, various team members' professions, practical examples of team-based medicine, medical ethics, medical safety, and the communication theory. It is primarily meant for freshman students (i.e., first-year students of the Schools of Pharmacy, Nursing, and Allied Health Sciences and third year students of the School of Medicine). The course was initiated during the last semester of SY2008. Part of the syllabus is shown in Table 4. In SY2009, the course became mandatory (worth one credit) for students of the Schools of Medicine and Allied Health Sciences, elective (semi-mandatory, worth one credit) for students of the School of Pharmacy, and optional for students of the School of Nursing (with a maximum number of student enrollment of about 1000). For the initial years the course is offered under various forms (mandatory, elective,

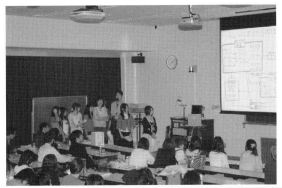
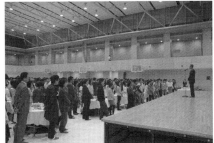
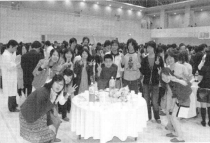

Fig. 5. All-Kitasato Team-Based Medical Drill (SY2008) (scene 2). Each of the 120 teams presents the outcome of its 2-day discussions. At the farewell party, the nine most distinguished teams receive awards

Table 3. Participation rate of students in the All-Kitasato Team-based Medical Drill (SY2008)
Time: May 1–2 (Thursday and Friday)
Venue: Sagamihara Campus

Participating school	No. of students in the targeted class	No. of participants	Attendance rate (%)
School of Pharmacy (4th-year students)	283	232	82.0
School of Medicine (5th-year students)	107	105	98.1
School of Nursing (4th-year students)	117	114	97.4
School of Allied Health Sciences (4th-year students; 3rd-year students for PT, OT, ST, HS)	423	397	93.9
College of Health and Hygienic Sciences (4th-year students; 3rd-year students for clinical laboratory course; 1st-year students for nondegree course)	269	262	97.4
Nursing School (3rd-year students)	40	39	97.5
Total	1239	1149	92.7

PT, physical therapy; OT, occupational therapy; ST, speech therapy; HS, health science
The number of attendees includes only those who were present on both days

Table 4. Outline of the syllabus of the Introduction to Team-based Medicine Lecture (SY2008)

Lecture no.	Content	Lecture topic
1	Introduction	Safe, high-quality medicine; the need for and value of team-based medicine
2	Outline of the health and welfare systems	Health and welfare systems of Japan and collaboration among systems; the people involved in the systems; comparison with other countries' systems; related topics
3	Understanding health professions—1	Educational system for each health profession; roles, functions, responsibilities, and positions in team-based medicine; examples of activities at various workplaces; related topics
4	Understanding health professions—2	As above
5	Understanding health professions—3	As above
6	Diseases and team-based medicine—1	Examples of team-based medicine and collaborative work among team members at actual medical sites; team dynamics, critical pass, clinical studies, among others
7	Diseases and team-based medicine—2	As above
8	Diseases and team-based medicine—3	As above
9	Medical ethics	Privacy and confidentiality; informed consent; notification of truth; birth and end-of-life stage; heredity and genes
10	Medical safety	Risk management in medicine
11	Communication theory	Communication among professionals; communication with patients; patient psychology; verbal and nonverbal communication; related topics
12	Advanced medicine and team-based medicine	Tailor-made medicine; gene therapy; regenerative medicine; related topics

optional) across schools; but in the coming years it will be made mandatory for all schools.

The course is offered remotely as a real-time two-way-dialogue style, online lecture for students of two colleges located in the university's Niigata Campus and Saitama Campus. For the time being, students of the two colleges only audit the lecture without receiving any credit. A total of 12 classes are scheduled for the fifth slot (16:20–17:50) of every Monday. At the university's Sagamihara Campus, students of the four health-related schools are randomly spread across four classrooms in one school building, which are all interconnected by a video-conferencing system for a real-time two-way-dialogue style lecture. Each classroom is attended to by an academic staff member who will assist, if necessary, for example, in allotting some additional time after the lecture for follow-up discussion to ensure the full educational effect of the lecture. The lecturers include the Vice President of the University, directors of the university-affiliated hospitals, directors of pharmaceutical and nursing departments of the university-affiliated hospitals, and other academic staff of the health-related schools in an omnibus style. Students are evaluated by the Educational Committee of each school in a comprehensive manner based on their term papers, class participation, and attendance records.

4 Implementation Arrangements for the Team-Based Medical Education Program

4.1 Implementation Arrangements and the Strategic Direction of the Whole University

4.1.1 Related Committees

4.1.1.1 Team-Based Medical Education Committee (Eight Members)

A committee for the whole university, the Team-Based Medical Education Committee, decides on the guiding principles and prepares the schedule, course contents, and curriculum of the entire program (i.e., the All-Kitasato Team-Based Medical Drill and the Introduction to Team-based Medicine lecture). About 10 meetings are held each year.

Chairperson: Vice President of the University. Members: Educational Committee chairperson of each school/college and Educational Committee chairperson of the college of Liberal Arts and Sciences.

4.1.1.2 Implementation Committee of Team-Based Medical Exercise (42 Members)

The Committee of Team-based Medical Exercise prepares the implementation plan, contents, and scenario (simulated cases) for the All-Kitasato Team-Based Medical Drill, whose participants number about 1200 students. This committee gives instructions and implements the exercise. About five or six meetings are held each year.

Chairperson: Vice President of the University. Members: members of the Team-Based Medical Education Committee (7), academic staff of each school/college (23), and the university's administrative staff members (11)—schools/colleges (5), Information Center (1), Education Center (5).

4.1.1.3 Facilitators for All-Kitasato Team-Based Medical Drill (~130 persons)

On the days of the exercise, one academic staff member is assigned to each of the 120 teams as its facilitator and assists the discussions of the student teams. Each school nominates its academic staff as the facilitators, whose total number is in proportion to the number of its participating students. Facilitators evaluate the students after the exercise.

4.1.2 Decision-Making Process Involving the Whole University

Decisions made by the two committees mentioned above are sent to the Committee of School Heads and then to the Board of Directors of the university for their respective approvals. After the decisions are approved, they are announced across the university.

4.2 Prior Education for Students, Academic Staff, and Administrative Staff

4.2.1 Team-Based Medical Education Forum (Four Times a Year)

Forums on team-based medicine and its education are held at the university's four campuses (i.e., Sagamihara, Shirokane, Niigata, Saitama) with the target audience the academic staff, administrative staff, and students. Information about the team-based medical education program at the university is disseminated. The Team-Based Medical Education Committee sponsors the forums.

4.2.2 Pre-Event Briefing for the Facilitators of All-Kitasato Team-Based Medical Drill (Four Times a Year)

At each of the university's four campuses, nominated facilitators (academic staff) are given pre-event briefing on the practical implementation procedures of the exercise and are requested to discuss issues as necessary. To avoid confusion and disorder at the small group discussions (SGD) of the 120 student teams, it is necessary to prepare a detailed manual for the exercise and make the facilitators fully understand it. The Team-Based Medical Education Committee sponsors the briefing.

4.2.3 Supporting and Cooperating Arrangements Within the University

All of the classes, including those at the schools other than the four health-related schools and also at the college of Liberal Arts and Sciences, are canceled during the 2 days of the All-Kitasato Team-Based Medical Drill. Buses are chartered and accommodations arranged for those students participating from remote campuses. The first-year students' curriculum at the college of Liberal Arts and

Sciences is adjusted for the students of the health-related schools such that they can take the Introduction to the Team-Based Medicine lecture at a common class slot while this lecture course is being properly incorporated into the curriculum of each school as a mandatory course or an elective (semi-mandatory) course.

5 Features and the Originality of the Program

- Practicing interprofessional team medicine requires, first, mutual understanding and respect among different health professions. Kitasato University, composed of four health-related schools and two colleges, produces graduates in as many as 14 health professions. This enables the university to conduct interprofessional education and to present its ideal model. The fact that the university prioritizes interprofessional education is another distinctive feature.
- Four hospitals affiliated with the university advocate patient-centered medical services and medicine built on collaboration (among and between health professionals, patients, and families). Hence, good appreciation for collaborative teamwork already exists in Kitasato. Underpinned by this spirit, the interprofessional education program enjoys active participation in and support from the whole university. Medical students also actively join.
- In particular, the All-Kitasato Team-Based Medical Drill has a remarkably high attendance rate (93% in 2008) despite its voluntary nature. This reflects not only interest and appreciation on the students' side toward team medicine but also commitment and enthusiasm on the academic staff's side.
- The university has developed GIOs and SBOs of its own and appreciates the importance of teamwork formation and mutual understanding among different disciplines. Stories of nine assignments (scenarios) are developed such that it can involve as many kinds of professions as possible.
- There is a plan for further development in the future (see Section 7).

6 Assessment of the Program

6.1 All-Kitasato Team-Based Medical Drill

A survey was conducted among the students on (1) the level of general satisfaction about the program (analyzed by school and by task) and (2) the degree of achievement of the seven SBOs in each of the nine tasks. Another survey was conducted among the academic staff (facilitators) regarding (1) the evaluation of the students' attitude and commitment, and (2) the assessment of the degree to which the SBOs were met by the students. The results indicated the following: (1) More than 90% of students replied that they were satisfied or slightly satisfied, suggesting that the program was generally well appreciated by the students. The level of satisfaction

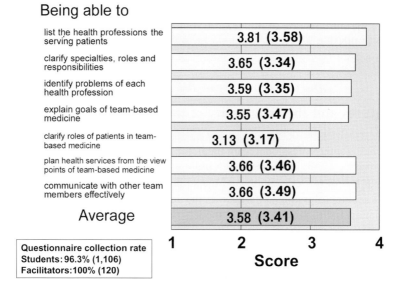

Fig. 6. Survey results on the degree of students' SBO achievement in the students' self-evaluation and by facilitators (SY2008). Assignments listed on the left side are the seven SBOs in Fig. 2. The degree of achievement is analyzed by a four-point scale. Figures show the facilitators' evaluation. Figures in parentheses show the results of the students' self-evaluation. Responses were collected from 96.3% of the students ($n = 1106$) and 100% of the facilitators ($n = 120$)

did not vary across schools but varied to some extent across tasks. It was therefore important to pay attention to these results when designing scenarios for the future. The level of satisfaction increased from 84% to 90% during the past three years. (2) The degree of achievement, measured by a four-point scale, varied from 3.17 (79%) on the level of understanding the role of patients in team medicine to 3.58 (90%) on the ability to list professions involved in serving patients holistically (Fig. 6). With the average being 3.58 (90%), the level of understanding about patients' roles in team medicine seems unimpressive. Students might have had difficulty understanding the questionnaire about the patients' roles. Interestingly, the facilitators' evaluation of the degree of SBO achievement shows the same tendency in the students' self-evaluation. The former indicates a degree of SBO achievement a little higher than the latter (Fig. 6).

6.2 Introduction to Team-Based Medicine Lectures

A comprehensive evaluation is done before giving credits to students by considering the attendance record, term paper, class participation, and the level of participation in discussions. A total of 1052 students registered for the program. Among them, an average of 874 students attended 10 lectures. A questionnaire survey with 17 questions was conducted at the final lecture, where 605 answers were collected. Major questions and typical answers are quoted as follows: (1) "Did the lecture contents interest you?" About 70% of students were positive, and 30% were negative. (2) Regarding the degree of achievement of SBOs, roughly 12% of students responded that they achieved more than 80% and 60% and 22% of students achieved 50%–79% and 22%–49%, respectively. For the multiple-choice question regarding what they gained from the lectures, 1377 responses were received, the breakdown of which is as follows: 68% of respondents appreciated the value and importance of team medicine, 46% understood other professions, 37% obtained new knowledge about team medicine, and 21% had an increased interest in practicing team medicine in the future. The results imply that first-year students do not necessarily understand team medicine well, which could be attributable to the organization of lectures. Lectures were delivered in an omnibus style, and each lecture might have been too intense for students to absorb. It seems that in the future it will be necessary to examine the entire case reports and their structure.

7 Development Plan

The future development of the Team-Based Medical Education Program depends on the effective collaboration and coordination between the four hospitals and the four schools and among the four hospitals themselves. Hence, discussions started in January 2008 among the three committees, as listed below.

- *Health Professions Education and Research Coordination Committee (HPERCC)*: Composed of a vice president, a board director, four school deans, two principals of the colleges, four hospital heads. Their purpose is to discuss the modalities of clinical training between hospitals and schools, and among hospitals.
- *Working Group of the HPERCC*: Composed of a vice president, educational chairpersons of schools, and training chairpersons of the hospitals. Its purpose is to develop an action plan in line with the decisions of the HPERCC. Together with the Team-Based Medical Education Committee (see below), the Working Group designs the educational content.
- *Team-Based Medical Education Committee* (see Section 4).

7.1 Team-Based Clinical Training

Students in lower classes (primarily first-year students) of health-related schools obtain basic knowledge about team medicine at the lecture Introduction to Team-Based Medicine. After that, they learn roles and responsibilities of their own professions through professional education of their respective schools. At the advanced classes (third to fifth year students), students participate in the All-Kitasato Team-Based Medical Drill and, further, appreciate team-based medicine through simulated case studies. The Team-Based Clinical Training Program is conducted as the next step (Fig. 3, step 3) to enhance practical capability. It was planned to start during 2009.

The Clinical Training Program is practical training conducted at four affiliated hospitals with actual working situations. However, it is impossible to provide this kind of training to all school students simultaneously owing to the large number of participants and curriculum constraints in each school. Hence, the training is done by rotation in small groups composed of limited numbers of students. The following training methods are under consideration.

- Participation in clinical training courses at hospitals that are already conducted as part of other schools' regular programs (for instance, students from other schools participate in the clinical clerkship program of the School of Medicine)
- Observatory participation in meetings on "critical path" at a hospital or experiencing team-based medicine such as preparation of a "path"
- Clinical training by diseases (in specialized centers) or by topic (palliative care, nutritional support, infection control, chemotherapy outpatient care at home, clinical trial studies, and so on)

To do this, effective and close coordination and planning is indispensable among hospitals and schools.

7.2 Project to Establish a Clinical Training Center for the Whole University

Kitasato University has multidisciplinary features (four health-related schools, two colleges, four affiliated hospitals, the Oriental Medicine Research Center, and so on), which is distinctive in Japan. To build on this advantage and to advance interprofessional team-based medicine, Kitasato University plans to establish a clinical training center. This system-wide university center will manage and coordinate cross-sectional clinical education activities among health-related schools conducted at four hospitals. To help this be realized, each hospital will establish an in-house clinical education center of its own and coordinate clinical training of the health-related schools. That is, these in-house centers will coordinate both professional training (vertical education) and cross-sectional/interprofessional training (lateral education) (Fig. 7).

The Oriental Medicine Research Center is affiliated with the university. It conducts basic research on herbal medicine and provides traditional medical services. It is unique, designated as a World Health Organization (WHO) Collaborating Center for Traditional Medicine. We plan to include this center in the team-based medical education program in the future.

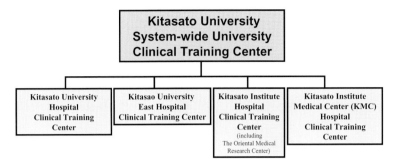

Fig. 7. Development plan for the System-wide Kitasato University Clinical Training Center

8 Conclusions

Medical services are becoming more sophisticated as life sciences advance. Epidemiological and demographic profiles are also changing drastically. Furthermore, social needs for holistic and humanized health care are ever increasing. Therefore, to respond effectively to these situations, interprofessional team-based medicine is of utmost importance. For instance, let us look at changes in the concept of drugs. Traditionally, drugs have been low-molecular-weight organic chemicals. Drugs, however, have evolved and include proteins and antibodies that are used for treatment; furthermore, they are incorporating the use of genes and cells. Finally, the advances in genome analysis are resulting in tailor-made and individualized treatments.

It is beyond the capacity of the health professions individually to respond to these newly emerging situations. Thus, team-based medicine is imperative to provide patient-centered, safer, high-quality health services. In fact, health services customarily are provided by teams. However, a paradigm shift is required from the *conventional* team-based, or shared, medicine (passive) to medicine developed through collaborative efforts—i.e., the *new* team-based, or collaborative, medicine (active). Education is urgently necessary to make this happen.

As mentioned above, Kitasato University has four health-related schools, two colleges, and four affiliated hospitals. It educates as many as 14 types of health-related specialist professionals. With these features, the university is well positioned to develop interprofessional team-based medicine. The university has been implementing distinctive team-based medical education program since 2006. In line with our future development plan, the university is determined to strengthen the program even further by making it a priority program.

Acknowledgment The authors sincerely thank Professor Hideomi Watanabe for his valuable comments and advice on team-based medical education as well as for the opportunity given by him to become a member of the Japan Interprofessional Working and Education Network (JIPWEN) and to prepare this chapter.

Becoming Interprofessional at Kobe University

Yumi Tamura[1], Yuichi Ishikawa[1], Peter Bontje[2], Taku Shirakawa[1], Hiroshi Andou[1], Ikuko Miyawaki[1], Kaori Watanabe[1], Yasushi Miura[1], Rei Ono[1], Kenichi Hirata[3], Midori Hirai[4], and Keiko Seki[1]

Summary

The importance of collaborative practice and its education have been widely reported globally and nationally. At a local level, staff members' experiences in the field after a natural disaster and their clinical work contributed significantly to the development of an interprofessional education/learning (IPE/L) program at Kobe University. From the first pilot classes in 2002, an IPE program evolved. This program is now fully integrated into the 4-year undergraduate curriculum at the Faculty of Health Sciences and into the 6-year curriculum of the School of Medicine. Student learning in this IPE/L program is interactive, experientially based, and predominantly conducted in interprofessional group settings.

During the first year students learn interprofessional basics in introductory subjects and, in addition, experience early exposure to clinical practice. During their second and third years, students' learning is applied to a range of concrete clinical areas related to health care provision in international in disaster health care.

[1]Kobe University Graduate School of Health Sciences, 7-10-2 Tomogaoka, Suma-ku, Kobe 654-0142, Japan
Tel./ Fax +81-78-796-4511
e-mail: ytbontje@kobe-u.ac.jp
[2]KIPEC (Kobe University Interprofessional Education for Collaborative Working Center), Kobe, Japan
[3]Kobe University, Graduate School of Medicine, Kobe, Japan
[4]Department of Pharmacology, Kobe University Hospital, Kobe, Japan

Correspondence to: Y. Tamura

Finally, students undertake interprofessional clinical practice, in interprofessional teams, at the patient/user level. Extracurricular activities, such as a student Interprofessional Work day and seminars and workshops held during an Interprofessional Work Week offer students additional opportunities to become interprofessional. These ongoing activities also disseminate knowledge and skills to educators from Kobe University and other educational institutions and professionals in clinical practice. The main tasks ahead are developing competencies for evaluation and evaluation methodologies for the IPE/L program. We also plan to develop an IPE/L component within the graduate school curriculum, particularly as a component of a course in International Activities for Health.

Key words Interprofessional curriculum · IPW-education · Learning together · Extracurricular activities · Student-led activity

The importance of collaborative practice and its education have been widely advocated globally and nationally. The World Health Organization (WHO) stressed the importance of "learning together" in 1987.[1] In 2003, the Organization for Economic Cooperation and Development (OECD) noted interchanges between different professions as a key competency. The National Institute of Medicine,[7] in 2003, identified that working in interdisciplinary teams is one of five competencies for health professions education. During the 1980s, White Papers from the Japanese Ministry of Health, Labor, and Welfare mentioned the importance of "team treatment" to encourage high-quality health care provision. However, the term "team treatment" was not defined, nor was it explained how it was to be practiced.

At a local level, research and development of Interprofessional Education/Learning (IPE/L) undertaken at Kobe University was instigated after staff experienced collaborative issues while providing health care following a natural disaster and from the wide range of clinical experience of the faculty. As an academic institution, it continuously formulates new questions to be answered and problems to be solved. This chapter gives an insight into how staff at the Faculty of Health Sciences grappled with such searching questions as "What is Interprofessional Work (IPW)?" "Why should we participate in IPE/L?" "What collaborative competencies should students acquire?" "What are appropriate teaching/learning methodologies?"

At this point, we point out that one of the conclusions reached was that acquiring collaborative competencies requires interactive, experiential learning. Therefore, we have adopted the term interprofessional education/learning to label our program. The first section of this chapter introduces the background and development of our IPE/L program. The second section outlines the actual program including some distinctive features such as the central role of students and tentative results. The third section briefly emphasizes our program's theoretical foundations. Finally, we outline conclusions from our program development experiences to date. We are honored to share our experiences. We hope that readers find this chapter a useful addition to their study of IPE/L or even to developing IPE/L in their own educational setting.

1 Road to IPE/L at Kobe University's Faculty of Health Sciences and Beyond

The first IPE/L classes were conducted in 2002 and went on to be developed into the IPE/L program presented here. Our IPE/L program was implemented during the 2007–2008 academic year with the implementation of a new curriculum. The IPE/L program is integrated across the 4 years of the health sciences' undergraduate curriculum (nursing, 80 students/year; medical laboratory technicians, 40 students/year; physical therapy, 20 students/year; occupational therapy, 20 students/year) and across the 6 years for students in the School of Medicine (100 students/year).

The heading of this section includes "and beyond" because the program reaches out to include students from Kobe Pharmaceutical University (from 2008) who participate in various aspects of the program. There are also extracurricular activities aimed at students and teaching staff at our and other educational institutions, as well as including clinicians.

1.1 Emergence of IPE/L in Relation to Kobe University

Various barriers to collaborative practice are mentioned throughout the literature. They include the use of inconsistent terminology, lack of understanding of professions, conflicts among health and medical professionals, and excessive specialization. We would also add that uniprofessional education fails to prepare health professionals adequately with IPW competencies. Since WHO highlighted the importance of "learning together" in 1987,[1] IPW education has been developing in such places as western Europe and North America. Yumi Tamura, who was a nurse in a Japanese hospital at that time, was one of the first to address these issues in Japan. She began to seriously question why health professionals from different fields cannot adequately collaborate for the benefit of their patients. After she experienced collaborative practice while abroad on Red Cross missions during the early 1990s, Tamura enrolled in the Interprofessional Health and Welfare Studies Master of Science course at London South Bank University, in part to address her searching question. During her thesis research, undertaken in Japan, Tamura found that even though students of different health professions were at times together in one classroom studying the same subject they were not "learning together." Upon return to Japan, Tamura, along with Kiyoko Ikegawa and Keiko Kudo, was invited to introduce the concept of "interprofessionalism" through a series of articles published in the journal *Quality Nursing*.[3]

Ten to fifteen years on, this publication serves as evidence that IPE/L is spreading in Japan through multiple channels and various initiatives. So, why is IPE/L attractive and seen to nurture professionals who can provide high-quality, safe, cost-effective health care? In answering this important question we first must consider the challenges of modern health care in Japan.

Progress in medicine has increased the variety of treatment options, some of which use highly advanced methods. In addition, greater demands are put on health care provision; and this progress, in turn, gives rise to ethical dilemmas (medical and bioethical). In addition, Japan's aging population coupled with a low birth rate puts added strains on financial and human resources. This situation gives rise to other important questions. First, who will be providing the treatment and care for patients in this changing environment? How will health care, rehabilitation, and home care systems be financially sustained in the future? To address the problems of a rapidly aging society, official policy promotes a shift to cheaper, more efficient (health) care in the community over institutionalized care. Such policy also recognizes that engagement in everyday life activities is conducive to helping the elderly and disabled people to maintain physical and cognitive function.

Recognizing the rights of health care users is seen as contributing to cost control while at the same time protecting human rights. Health care workers not only work in traditional environments such as hospitals but increasingly provide services in patients' homes and in community-based facilities.

To meet the users' needs, a variety of new health professions and specializations have evolved. The number of health care workers, particularly nurses, care attendants, home helpers, and rehabilitation professionals, are increasing at a rapid rate. This situation increases the risk of fragmentation because communication among health care workers and coordination of service provision has become more complex. Finally, all too often health care recipients fall ill or sustain serious injuries or permanent disabilities, and some even die owing to accidents. Adequate collaboration among health care workers can prevent many of such accidents from happening. In short, health care workers face the challenge of providing safe, trustworthy, patient-centered services so people can receive quality health care services with peace of mind.

Interprofessional work (IPW) has been identified as one efficient way to promote safe, cost-effective, patient-centered services. IPW does this by preventing fragmentation of care, ensuring that patient needs are not overlooked, and by including the patient and his or her family as important team members who become involved in their health care.

Natural disasters can serve in part to highlight the importance of IPW. Unfortunately, Kobe is probably best known for the Great Hanshin-Awaji earthquake, which occurred in the early morning hours of January 17, 1995. Kobe University Hospital was damaged in the disaster, but it continued to offer medical treatment as the core hospital in the disaster region. Hospital staff responded to the needs of survivors of the earthquake by opening temporary clinics that provided some of the most important medical treatment in the area. This response required instant planning, flexibility, and above all coordination of activities and resources. Together with local therapists, the university's occupational and physical therapy faculty pitched in with immediate relief efforts, such as transporting survivors and assisting in the distribution of basic necessities in shelters. During these activities, the rehabilitation professionals became aware that exercise and activities for disabled people and the frail elderly were not being provided in the shelters. In response, they formed teams and introduced "home" rehabilitation in shelters. When these older and disabled people moved into temporary housing, the rehabilitation professionals became aware that temporary housing was all but barrier-free. Together with the authorities responsible they helped make these temporary houses accessible to people with disabilities.

Hyogo Prefecture has suffered from severe floods in its northern areas, and Kobe University dispatched interprofessional medical support teams (consisting of medical doctors, nurses, and pharmacologists). After receiving instructions from city hall, one team was charged with the responsibility of providing health checks in a temporary shelter together with a Red Cross team. Another team went into an affected community, providing health care and assisting people in cleaning up their homes.

Interprofessional teams have also been active in Aceh, Indonesia, in the aftermath of the tsunami in 2004 and some two years later in 2006 following an earthquake on the island of Java. In both cases, the interprofessional teams from Kobe University who responded to the disasters were made up of professionals well-matched to the local needs and planned activities. Collaboration with Indonesian partner universities made these missions possible and shaped the formation of the teams (two medical doctors, a nurse, a pharmacist, and a clerk were dispatched to Aceh and a pediatrician, a dietician, and a physical therapist to Java).

In conclusion, from their experiences, the staff at Kobe University came to understand that cooperation among organizations and collaboration among health professionals is essential for promoting patient-focused safe health care. We also regard IPW as contributing to cost-effective high-quality health care. However, IPW is still evolving and is not easy to implement. Consequently, it is necessary to foster students' and health workers' collaborative skills. In this respect we have adopted the WHO policy that states, "joint learning can lead to changes in attitudes of medical service workers, establishment of common values and other norms, organization of teams, resolution of problems, fulfillment of needs, and changes in practices and health professions."[1] It is clearly important for students who are training to be health professionals in diverse fields to study and learn together to develop sound competencies required for patient-centered IPW. Based on this concept, the faculty committed itself to set about developing an IPE/L curriculum that is fully integrated into the curriculum of both health sciences and medicine curricula. In combination with extracurricular activities, IPW graduate research and education is currently being further developed. We aim to create wide ripple effects whereby our IPE/L education ultimately influences and facilitates IPW for the benefit of all health care recipients.

1.2 *Developing and Implementing IPE/L at Kobe University*

Trends and challenges in health care and experiences in disaster relief work highlighted the need for education to foster collaborative competencies in students who will become future health care providers. IPE/L was introduced into our agenda by Yumi Tamura, who joined the health sciences faculty in 2001 and conducted the first classes introducing IPW in 2002. In combination with faculty and curriculum development activities, this initiative grew into a program that included the four professions of the health sciences faculty and students from the School of Medicine. Opportunities for integrating IPE/L into the curriculum arose, with the planning for a reformed curriculum to be implemented during the 2007–2008 academic year.[1] What's more, given the increasing competition[2] between universities in Japan, development of IPE/L was adopted as one of the special features of the Faculty of Health Sciences' profile.

We have chosen to use a tree to depict our mission statement (Fig. 1), which was adopted in 2004–2005 as part of our Universities Profiling Project. At the tree-

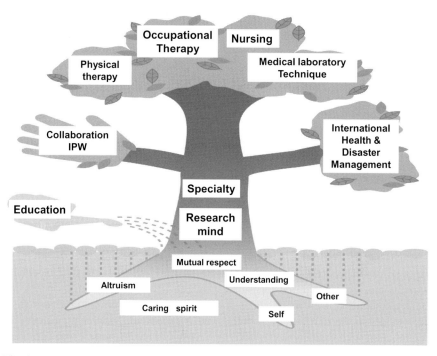

Fig. 1. Tree of Kobe University's Faculty of Health Sciences' mission statement. *IPW*, interprofessional work

---

[1] This coincided with educational reforms associated with state universities, such as Kobe University, becoming educational institutions legally independent from the Ministry of Education, Culture, Sports, Science, and Technology in 2004.

[2] In Japan, aging of society is not only caused by longer life expectancy but also by a low birth rate of approximately 1.3. Recruitment of high school graduates to fill university seats is becoming highly competitive.

top are the four professions' undergraduate courses leading to qualifications such as physical therapists (PTs), occupational therapists (OTs), nurses (NSs) and medical laboratory technicians (MTs). To the right is International Health and Disaster Health Management, which is another aspect of our profile. To the left is the branch called Collaboration. The trunk and roots symbolize values important to the future of our students as health professionals. Last but not least, our education provides the nutrients for growth.

In 2003, an IPE/L subcommittee was formed within the Faculty Development Committee. This IPE/L subcommittee studied and developed the IPE/L program. Masters students participated in several research projects addressing issues related to IPW and IPE/L. In addition to student research activities, the faculty undertook research on the IPE/L classes that were conducted at that time. For example, we published research findings about the educational use of menus as a metaphor for IPW. We found that "presumed to be inexperienced" first-year students demonstrated that they were able to conceptualize interprofessional collaboration and identify professional values and issues involved in making team treatment work.[4]

Various faculty-development seminars and workshops were organized with invited international scholars of IPW and IPE/L, such as Tony Leiba (London South Bank University) in 2003, Hugh Barr (CAIPE and Westminster University), John Gilbert (InterEd and the University of British Colombia) in 2005, Tony Leiba again in 2006 and in 2007 together with Jenny Weinstein (London South Bank University) and Helena Low (CAIPE/L). Louise Nasmith (the University of British Colombia) presented in 2008. Japanese scholars such as Gunma University's Dr. Watanabe (editor of this book), Dr. Naoki Saji (Himeji Brain and Heart Center) in 2008, and Dr. Yuko Takeda (Mie University) in 2007 presented topics relating to collaborative issues as well as to teaching/learning methods for IPW and IPE/L.

We also drew on expertise from international bodies. Coauthor Yuichi Ishikawa, currently Dean of the Faculty of Health Sciences, was present at the kick-off event in 2006 of InterEd (the International Association for Interprofessional Education and Collaborative Practice). Ishikawa is a current board member of InterEd; and InterEd's collaboration with the WHO study group on interprofessional education was an additional source of expertise on which we drew. Another important international resource was CAIPE (Centre for the Advancement of Interprofessional Education).

1.3 Conclusion

Trends in medicine and health care and local experiences clearly demonstrated the need for IPE/L. We have adopted the following definitions of IPW and IPE/L.
- IPW, or interprofessional work—collaborative teamwork by various health professionals for people who need health care and to care for the elderly and

disabled people in their community (definition from the Kobe University Faculty of Health Sciences).
- IPE/L, or interprofessional education/learning—occurs when two or more professions learn with, from, and about each other to improve collaboration and the quality of care (definition adopted from CAIPE)

Educational reforms provided the opportunity to develop an IPE/L program that is fully integrated in the undergraduate curriculum. Like other IPE/L initiatives presented in this book, we started from scratch. IPE/L started modestly within a nursing course in 2002 but grew to include all four professions at the Faculty of Health Sciences in 2004. The IPE/L program is now integrated across the 4-year undergraduate curriculum. The School of Medicine joined the program in 2006. An IPW component will be developed for medical students' clinical affiliations in their fifth and sixth years, too. As of 2007, students from Kobe Pharmaceutical University have been able to join parts of the curriculum if they wish, and currently a maximum of 50 of them opt to do so each year.

2 Introduction to the 4-Year Program

The IPW competencies the students learn cover collaboration among health professionals and cooperation among organizations. The learning of IPW, which is required to address issues of modern medicine and health and home care is incorporated into the curriculum in both general and specialized courses. There are also extracurricular activities. The IPE/L program has the following educational goals for the students.

1. Understand the core concept of "interprofessional."
2. Understand and respect the roles of different health professions.
3. Acquire knowledge and skills that can be shared across professional borders (skill mix).
4. Understand meanings and values of collaboration and develop a positive attitude toward collaboration.
5. Acquire skills required for collaboration (leadership, team organization, problem identification and problem-solving abilities, proposal writing, coordination, communication skills) and demonstrate these skills in practice.
6. Appreciate the reforms needed in health sciences, medical care and welfare from an IPW perspective.

2.1 Outline of the IPE/L Program in the Undergraduate Curriculum

Kobe University's IPE/L program commences during the first term of the first year with an introduction to interprofessional work and modern medicine and bioethics.

At the end of the first term there is early exposure to clinical practice, wherein students from Kobe Pharmaceutical University participate (they study modern medicine and bioethics via e-learning).

In the Faculty of Health Sciences, all second-year students study international and disaster health care. During the third year they take part in IPW exercises in international and disaster health care activities. Fourth-year students in both health sciences and the medical faculties take clinical-based IPW training, which addresses health/medical problems from an IPW perspective in the context of a clinical practice.[3]

Figure 2 depicts the above IPE/L program. Please note at the top left that the program includes the fifth and sixth years of the medical students' curriculum. We are now considering how medical students can further learn IPW competencies during their internship.

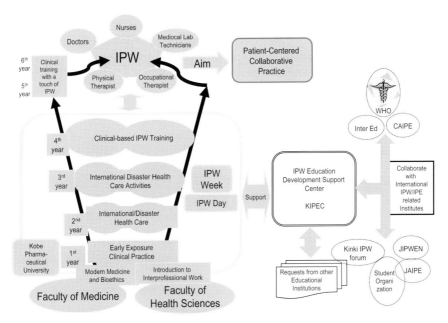

Fig. 2. Systematic interprofessional education/learning (IPE/L) for collaborative competencies. *WHO*, World Health Organization; *Inter Ed*, interprofessional education; *CAIPE*, Centre for the Advancement of Interprofessional Education; *KIPEC*, Kobe University Interprofessional Education for Collaborative Work Center; *JIPWEN*, Japan Interprofessional Working and Education Network; *JAIPE*, Japan Association for Interprofessional Education

---

[3] Please note that as the IPE/L program was implemented in 2007 this interprofessional clinical practice will be first offered during the 2010–2011 academic year. The plan is that in 2011–2012 this will be scenario-based problem-based learning. If all goes well, this clinical practice will be conducted in clinical institutions with the cooperation of patients in 2011–2012.

2.2 Outlines of the Various Subjects

Currently the IPE/L program is in its third year of implementation. Here we outline the IPE/L program by describing the subjects that have been implemented in the program to date.

2.2.1 Introduction to Interprofessional Work

First year, first term; Faculty of Health Sciences only; 15 sessions × 2 hours, 1 credit; compulsory

The introduction to IPW provides students indispensable knowledge and skills for IPW. They work in interprofessional teams, but are also encouraged to explore each profession's specialty. The first half of this subject deals with how to build and maintain interpersonal relationships based on knowing oneself and on understanding others, as well as acquiring communication skills. Applying the principle of learning-by-doing to practice, much practice is included and this part ends with meeting and communicating with persons with aphasia.

In the latter half of this subject, students learn, in experiential ways, to work in interprofessional teams. The content of the course is based on team building, and at the end of this part groups create and present "images of professionals" (typically in pictures).

2.2.2 Modern Medicine and Bioethics

First year, first term; Faculties of Health Sciences and Medicine; 15 sessions × 2 hours, 1 credit; compulsory

In an omnibus-style, faculty and guest lecturers cover a wide range of topics regarding modern medicine and bioethics, with the purpose of having students acquire an understanding of the essence of medicine. This subject explores issues related to bioethics and law; patient rights; progress of medicine; safety of medical treatment; meeting society's demand for trustworthy, high-level, cost-effective treatments and rehabilitation; health care workers' conduct; and psychological care and support. These issues affect all profession(al)s, and no single profession(al) is expected to be able to deal with these issues alone. Although the content of the course is taught in a traditional lecture-type setting, learning also takes place in interprofessional groups. The groups grapple with these issues using menus as a metaphor for team work. The interprofessional groups finally present what they learned about the meaning and value of IPW. The experiences hitherto are that the groups demonstrate an understanding of the role of one's own and other professions, the position of the patient (patient-centered teams), team processes (i.e., influences of status and hierarchy), and so forth.

2.2.3 Early Exposure Clinical Practice

First year, first term; Kobe University Faculties of Health Sciences and Medicine (compulsory), Kobe Pharmaceutical University (elective); 3 days/1 week, 1 credit

During a 1-week course (Fig. 3), undertaken at the end of the first term, students visit a clinical setting. As participants in interprofessional teams, they observe and experience the various professions' roles and gain a greater understanding of how professionals work together for the patients. The interprofessional teams include students from Kobe Pharmaceutical University.

Day 1 is for orientation, and invited ex-patients talk about their experiences with health care and give their thoughts and expectations they have of health professional students (Fig. 3). On day 2, 3 or 4 students spend one day on interprofessional teams in one of a wide variety of health care and welfare facilities. Or they study their own profession in uniprofessional groups. Day 5 is at the university; and during the morning, the interprofessional teams discuss and summarize what they learned from the visits. In the afternoon, the groups share their learning through presentations. In addition to learning from an interprofessional perspective, students are stimulated to learn about health workers' attitudes and conduct, health care's mission from a societal perspective, ethics, humanity, and so forth through reflection on their individual experiences.

Day 1	Day 2	Day 3	Day 4	Day 5
All together (310 students) Orientation. Listen to and learning from (ex-) patients' experiences and expectations	Joint clinical practice *6-7students from more than three professionals per group *22 groups *22 hospitals /institutions	Joint clinical practice *6-7students from more than three professionals per group *23 groups *23 hospitals /institutions	Clinical practice within own department	All together (310 students) Presentation of learning from joint clinical practice (modified menus) Semiformal BBQ party
	Clinical practice within own department	Clinical practice within own department		

Fig. 3. Early exposure to clinical practice

2.2.4 International and Disaster Health Care

Second year, second term; Faculty of Health Sciences only; 15 sessions × 2 hours, 1 credit; compulsory

The study of international and disaster health care starts with the north–south health gap, including the causes and background influences. Students proceed to learn about the main tasks in international health and health care in times of disaster, including applicable frameworks. The main methods of learning are lectures and group discussions, where students share what they have learned and discuss it with students from other professions.

2.2.5 International and Disaster Health Care Activities

Third year, first term; Faculty of Health Sciences only; 7, 5 sessions × 4 hours, 1 credit; compulsory

Building on the more theoretical learning during the second-year "International and Disaster Health Care" course, the students explore and/or experience a sample of relevant health care activities, such as general effects of disasters and how people respond following a disaster, polio vaccination, triage, and strategies in times of disaster (Médecins Sans Frontières). In interprofessional groups, students discuss case studies to further their understanding and develop IPW competencies, including communication skills, team building, and problem identification and problem-solving skills.

2.3 Evidence: Results and Evaluation

Carpenter and Dickinson[5] gave an overview of some research evidence making a case for interprofessionalism but also pointed out that much more research is needed. A Cochrane review by Reeves et al.[6] concluded that the quality of available research was insufficient to state that IPE/L is effective and to understand the key features of IPE/L. However, we are encouraged that some studies demonstrated that IPE/L resulted in improved cooperative work and the provision of better care from these professionals.

As for evaluating our local results, for the time being we draw on students' feedback on the various subjects and the administration of an IPW readiness measure called RIPLS (Readiness of Health Care Students for Interprofessional Learning).[7] Next, we present some tentative results. Some of them were presented at the 18th Net07 Networking for Education in Health Care conference in Cambridge in 2007 and the All Together for Better Health II conference in Stockholm in 2008.

The RIPLS consists of three subscales (total 19 items): Teamwork and Collaboration (items 1–9); Professional Identity (items 10–16); Roles and Responsibility (items 17–19). Students rate on a Likert-type four-point scale how they feel about the items' statements, from "strongly agree" to "strongly disagree." We adopted RIPLS for two reasons: (1) Assessing changes in readiness for IPE/L seems a valid evaluation at the undergraduate level; and (2) we judged the RIPLS's items to be relevant and reflective of our local situation. The Japanese translation of the question items resulted in a culturally appropriate version, but reliability studies have yet to be performed. RIPLS was administered at the beginning and end of each term in 2005, 2006, and 2007 and also after clinical practice in 2007 (which took place after the end-of-term examinations).

Furthermore, we have data from student questionnaires that the university routinely conducts on all the subjects in the curriculum. These questionnaires ask students for their opinion about each subject (e.g., level of difficulty, quality of teachers' instructions, perceived usefulness to their professional future).

We arrived at some conclusions regarding the above data.

- Students of nursing and occupational therapy have generally similar views and are most ready and willing to engage in collaboration; however, in one evaluation fewer than 50% of medical laboratory technique students saw IPW skills as necessary. In another evaluation only one-third of the medical laboratory technician and physical therapy students saw IPE as beneficial for communication between clients and professionals.
- Students found interprofessional learning useful to their future and would like to have more of these learning opportunities.
- Students become more able to understand their own and others' professional views.
- According to the students, establishing effective teams takes time. They also found that students of medicine should participate in the IPE program.
- Scores demonstrated increased IPW readiness after clinical practice, but that increase was not evident (statistically) after classroom learning.
- In 2008, the subject "Introduction to IPW" was commended because students rated of highest among all subjects in the health sciences curriculum.

These results have helped shape the IPE program for the new curriculum. The results supported the inclusion of students of medicine, inspired measures to deal with restrictions imposed by an auditorium-style classroom, and faculty development activities (e.g., a training weekend, which includes students, on facilitation techniques).

2.4 Extracurricular Activities: IPW Day and IPE/L Circle

We believe that clinical practice is the best place to learn collaboration because it directly practices "working together." However, there is no clinical practice during the second and third years. The second and third year international and health disaster health care subjects are also without medical students. Therefore, we have implemented extracurricular activities in which second- and third-year students are active. For example, an annual IPW Week is to be organized by faculty with support of students (the first IPW week was held 2–7 November 2009). Another annual event, the IPW Day is planned, prepared, and conducted by the students. In 2008, we provided them with funding to invite Canadian students Jason Hoffman and Steven Nickerson, who talked about students as change agents of IPW. Students from Saitama, Gunma, and Tsukuba (their interprofessional education programs are outlined elsewhere in this book) also attended. This has led to the formation of a student IPW Club at Kobe University, and currently students are exploring possibilities of establishing a national IPW student network. The student circle has recently been involved in seminars and study meetings concerning facilitation.

Since 2003, we have organized an annual study meeting, usually including a seminar/symposium-style session and a workshop. The persistent feedback has been that the audience wanted more time. Therefore, from the autumn of 2009 we plan for an IPW week with a seminar and a workshop on separate days. The purpose is to disseminate IPW and IPE/L to the Faculty of Health Sciences, other health care educational institutions, and the clinical arenas. Although IPW week activities touch on the need for IPW and IPE/L and what they are, the main focus is on how IPW and IPE/L can be achieved. Therefore, learning is experience-based; and active participation in various forms (e.g., group work, play, scenario-based situated learning, discussion, and presentation) is a central feature.

2.5 Additional Activities

A regional collaboration since 2006 between health science faculties of Osaka University and Kyoto University resulted in a regularly scheduled Kinki Team Treatment (in Japanese: *chi-mu iryou*) Forum and publication of the *Kinki Journal of Interprofessional Care*.

More recently, Ishikawa and Tamura have participated as board members of the national organizations Japan Interprofessional Working and Education Network (JIPWEN) and the Japanese Association for Interprofessional Education (JAIPE).

2.6 Conclusion

The IPE/L program that has been developed and integrated into the undergraduate curriculum started from several modest classes introducing undergraduate students to IPW in 2002. Learning of IPW has some theoretical components, but it unfolds most fully in interprofessional group work and in clinical practice. It is also applied to international and disaster health care. Most of the learning requires active participation, and skills training takes place in the classroom and in clinical settings. Extracurricular activities offer extra opportunities for working and learning together when medical students and students from Kobe Pharmaceutical University do not have IPE/L courses. Engaging in these extracurricular activities also hones students' project management skills. Finally, these extracurricular activities function to demonstrate to students the ripple effects IPE/L may have beyond themselves and their universities. We hope that our students will become role models and facilitators in the development of IPW and IPE/L in various medical institutions and health and home care settings.

One important scholarly challenge is to develop evaluation methodologies that enable us to verify that students indeed acquire IPW competencies which contribute to the provision of high-quality, safe, trustworthy, patient-centered services.

Information on our IPE/L program, including videos of workshops, seminars, and some lectures, can be accessed at the website of Kobe University Interprofessional Education for Collaborative Work Center (KIPEC) via: http://www.edu.kobe-u.ac.jp/fhs-gpipw/.

3 Theoretical and Educational Foundations

Interprofessional work is practiced in a wide variety of settings; thus, different collaborative knowledge, skills, and attitudes may be more or less important. Students may acquire necessary collaborative competencies in a variety of ways. This may depend on what is required, but it also depends on personal preferences for learning. These aspects were considered when we designed our IPE/L program. At the undergraduate level, most students enter directly from high school. For many of them, participating in the IPE/L program involves a transition because in this program they are regarded as subjects who are active agents of their learning with an emphasis on experiential learning, clinical practice, and extracurricular activities.

At a more fundamental level, "learning together to work together" is the basic idea underpinning the design of our IPE/L program. The book *Going Interprofessional* by Leathard[8] is among the most influential literature offerings for our IPE/L program. Most learning takes place in interprofessional groups, so students share their learning and develop IPW competencies. Given the importance we attach to mutual understanding and communication skills, we like to talk of "learning from each other about each other." We also regard experiential learning as conducive to developing skills such as setting common goals, decision making, resolution of problems, developing common values and norms, organization of teams, and role allocation, among others. Finally, the variety of subjects, classroom and clinical practice learning, and, for some, the extracurricular activities show the students how different settings require different emphasis in IPW competencies.

Other important theoretical and educational foundations are the following.

- Adult-learning theories[9] and reflective learning.[10] We attach importance to these points to prepare students for lifelong learning and for those who wish to develop IPW in their practices.

- Team-building skills and facilitation techniques. These attributes are not only for students' futures as lifelong learners and leaders but also for faculty members to develop didactic skills appropriate to the teaching/learning methodologies of the IPE/L program.[11]
- The 3P model of presage–process–product as one tool to inform the development of the IPE/L program.[12]
- Although still developing, interprofessional competencies such as the collaborative capacities formulated by Barr.[13]
- User involvement to promote client-centeredness.
- Communication and social skills.
- Sociology and psychology of working in teams and group behavior.

4 Conclusion

From our tentative attempts to introduce IPW to nursing students, an IPE/L program has evolved that is now in its third year of implementation. We are currently endeavoring to implement the IPE/L program in the fourth to sixth years of the curricula. Developing and implementing this program required a pioneering spirit, with our efforts being supported by national and international experts and research grants. Many teachers collaborated and participated in faculty and curriculum development activities, with 10–12 teachers forming a core group to propel developments forward. We take pride in that the School of Medicine and Kobe Pharmaceutical University asked to join the IPE/L program. The establishment of a student IPW circle was beyond our expectations.

Despite our success, there are still hurdles to be overcome and hills to be climbed. Developing a student evaluation protocol is one major task. The evaluation of teachers' perceptions and the whole project are also on the agenda. Good evaluation is important as it can identify the students' and the program's strengths and weaknesses. Such information can inform the tasks ahead of continuously developing our IPE/L program.

Teachers' didactic and facilitation skills may also be further polished to reach a higher level appropriate to the theoretical and philosophical underpinnings of the IPE/L. Masters of Science and doctoral courses and research are currently being developed in the International Health Department of our graduate school. We are envisioning research and study with IPW and IPE/L dimensions of international health and disaster medicine and management. Such research may also further inform the development of the IPE/L program at the undergraduate level.

In Japan, White Papers of the Ministry of Health started mentioning *chi-mu iryou*, which translates as team treatment, as far back as the 1980s. However, the term was not adequately explained (it certainly was not patient centered), nor was there any urgency or ideas of how team treatment was to be taught to the students. In reality, nothing much changed; and to the best of our knowledge, there were no studies or analyses that accounted for this state of affairs. Perhaps it was because collaboration was seen as something commonplace, and people believed that they worked collaboratively. This state of affairs was to change, however, and team treatment became a buzzword around the year 2000.

The faculty of Health Sciences at Kobe University started IPE/L in 2002. Whereas global and national contexts made the case for IPE/L in general, IPE/L here has a local flavor. The university attaches much importance to contributing to health management during and after natural disasters. In regard to students' futures as health professionals, the IPE/L program attaches much importance to mutual respect and understanding between professionals and patient centeredness based on communication. We have designed an interactive, experientially based learning program that we believe nurtures health professionals and that can provide cost-efficient, safe, high-quality patient-centered health care.

Acknowledgments We thank the guest lecturers mentioned above and all staff from the Kobe University Faculty of Health Sciences and School of Medicine for their contributions. Many of the developmental activities, including inviting the guest lecturers and the establishment of the Kobe University Interprofessional Education for Collaborative Work Center (KIPEC), were made possible with the "Distinctive University Education Support Program (Good Practice)" educational development grant awarded for the period beginning in the autumn of 2007 and lasting to the spring of 2010.

References

1. WHO (1987) Learning together to work together for health. Geneva: World Health Organization
2. Institute of Medicine (2003) Health professions education: a bridge to quality. National Academies Press, Washington DC
3. Tamura Y, Kudo K, Ikekawa K (1998) What is Inter-professional? Rawson D's conceptual mode. Qual Nurs 4:1032–1040
4. Tamura Y, Bontje P, Nakata Y, et al (2005) Can one eat collaboration? Menus as metaphors of interprofessional collaboration. J Interprof Care 19:215–222
5. Carpenter J, Dickinson H (2008) Interprofessional education and training. Policy Press, Bristol
6. Reeves S, Zwarenstein M, Goldman J, et al (2008) Interprofessional education: effects on professional practice and health care outcomes. Cochrane Database Syst Rev (1):CD002213
7. Parsell G, Bligh J (1999) The development of a questionnaire to assess the readiness of health care students for interprofessional learning (RIPLS). Med Educ 33:95–100
8. Leathard A (1994) Going inter-professional: working together for health and welfare. Routledge, London
9. Knowles MS (1990) The adult learner: a neglected species. Gulf Publications, Houston
10. Schön DA (1987) Educating the reflective practitioner: toward a new design for teaching and learning in the professions. Jossey-Bass, San Francisco
11. Hori K, Kato A, Karube T (2007) Team building (in Japanese). Nikkei Books, Tokyo
12. Freeth D, Reeves S (2004) Learning to work together: using the presage, process, product (3P) model to highlight decisions and possibilities. J Interprof Care 18:43–56
13. Barr H (1998) Competent to collaborate: towards a competency-based model for interprofessional education. J Interprof Care 12:181–187

Interprofessional Education Initiatives at Gunma University: Simulated Interprofessional Training for Students of Various Health Science Professions

Hatsue Ogawara[1], Tomoko Hayashi[2], Yasuyoshi Asakawa[3], Kiyotaka Iwasaki[4], Tamiko Matsuda[2], Yumiko Abe[1], Fusae Tozato[4], Takatoshi Makino[2], Hiromitsu Shinozaki[2], Misako Koizumi[2], Takako Yasukawa[3,5], and Hideomi Watanabe[3]

Summary

The School of Health Sciences (the "School") of the Gunma University has a mandate to train and produce advanced, high-quality health professionals. To enhance collaboration among health professionals and to overcome the fragmented nature of specialized medicine, the School has developed a curriculum based fundamentally on holistic medicine and interprofessional work (IPW). The major advantage of the curriculum lies in its training program—simulated interprofessional training—where students work in groups and undergo a series of activities, including

---

[1]Department of Laboratory Science, School of Health Sciences, Gunma University, Maebashi, Japan
[2]Department of Nursing, School of Health Sciences, Gunma University, Maebashi, Japan
[3]Department of Physical Therapy, School of Health Sciences, Gunma University, 3-39-15 Showa, Maebashi, 371-8511, Japan
Tel. +81-27-220-8945; Fax +81-27-220-8999
e-mail: hidewat@health.gunma-u.ac.jp
[4]Department of Occupational Therapy, School of Health Sciences, Gunma University, Maebashi, Japan
[5]Department of Internal Medicine, Seirei Hamamatsu General Hospital, Hamamatsu, Japan

Correspondence to: H. Watanabe

All members belong to the Interprofessional Education Committee of Gunma University (IPEC-GU)

group discussions, clinical training at facilities, general meetings, and reporting. This "teamwork training" is the core subject of the education. Its concept is first shared and discussed during the first year of the curriculum, and training is introduced to the third-year students from all departments of the School. All academic staff help implement the training in cooperation with approximately 20 external health care facilities. The training is evaluated every year, and both students and academic staff have evaluated it positively. This "teamwork training" has been in practice for 9 years now. As medical knowledge has expanded and technology advanced, changes have taken place in IPW at clinical settings. To respond to this, deliberate efforts are being made, including: (1) use of updated case scenarios; (2) participation of students from the School of Medicine; and (3) networking for interprofessional education with external medical facilities and other universities.

Key words Simulated interprofessional training · Health sciences · Networking for IPE

1 Profile and Mission of Gunma University

Gunma University (the "University") consists of four faculties: Education, Social and Information Studies, Medicine, and Engineering. The School of Health Sciences (the "School") was established in 1996 under the Faculty of Medicine in addition to the existing School of Medicine. The School has four departments: Nursing, Laboratory Sciences, Physical Therapy, and Occupational Therapy. The School provides an undergraduate program (4 years), a master's course (2 years in the first term of the postgraduate school), and a doctorate course (3 years in the second term of the postgraduate school).

The University, aiming at producing graduates who would serve the society, has been promoting practical education and operational research founded on basic science. The intent of this concept is to respond to evolving social needs and demands. Since the beginning of the 21st century, however, a variety of new and unprecedented issues have arisen owing to rapid social and environmental changes. Under this social context, the University has developed a new mission statement that advocates producing graduates who are competent, capable of conducting advanced scientific research at the international level, able to grasp the essence of issues without being affected by superficiality, courageous enough to approach new issues innovatively, and well qualified to deliver quality services to society.

2 Background and Goals of the IPE Program

Health care services have become highly specialized owing to the rapid progress and advances in modern medicine. Such specialized services require involvement of a diverse range of medical professionals much more than traditional health workers, physicians, and nurses. In view of an epidemiological change, attributable to the aging of the population, industrial structural changes, and social demands for safe, high-quality medical services, highly specialized professionals play essential roles in health care provision, including preventive care and physical therapy. However, there is concern that under these circumstances health professionals have increasingly developed narrow views, focusing only on organs and aspects of a disease or disorder in which they have specialized. To minimize this adverse effect, a team educational approach, interprofessional education (IPE), is of utmost importance as it enables functional integration of all specialized skills into patient-centered care.

Interprofessional education is a challenge common to all educational institutions of health professions. The School has been providing IPE for 9 years. The IPE program is a regular subject, mandatory for all third-year students in the School. It is held every Friday morning for 2 hours (one lesson lasts 2 hours) throughout the year (a total of 45 lessons). It also includes 2-day clinical training (equivalent to 10 lessons) and a 1-day debriefing meeting (equivalent to 5 lessons). In 2007, however, the class was held for 4 hours a week, concentrated during the first term, as requested by students. The curricula up to the academic year 2007 are explained in this chapter.

The program's goals were as follows.

- Educational goals of "teamwork training," a core program in IPE
    - Experience being part of a health care team (the spirit of interprofessional work)
    - Learn about interprofessional work in clinical practice (the skills of interprofessional work)
- Other effects derived from the IPE program
    - Interaction through group work among students across departments
    - Development of professionalism, leading to awareness of social responsibility
    - Collaboration among academic staff across departments through the joint program management

3 Educational Content of the IPE Program

3.1 Importance of IPE in the School of Health Sciences

The School of Health Sciences consists of the departments of Nursing (80 students), Laboratory Sciences (40 students), Physical Therapy (20 students), and Occupational Therapy (20 students). Since its establishment in 1996, it has been contributing to the IPE program the principle of holistic medicine. Figure 1 outlines the IPE program in the 4-year undergraduate program. First-year students learn the details

Department / Academic year	Nursing	Laboratory Science	Physical Therapy	Occupational Therapy
I	**Liberal subjects** Holistic medicine/Teamwork studies Interprofessional work			
II	**Advanced basic subjects**			
III	**Teamwork clinical training** **Expertise subjects · Expertise clinical training**			
IV	**Expertise clinical training** **Research for the graduation thesis**			

Fig. 1. Positioning of interprofessional education (IPE) in the School of Health Sciences

and value of interprofessional work in lectures. Two subjects are covered: Holistic Medicine/Teamwork Studies, a mandatory basic science course (during the first term) and Interprofessional Work Overview, an elective general education course (second term; there are 15 lessons on each subject. Built on the professional expertise acquired during the second year, third-year students participate in teamwork training, which is mandatory; the training is provided over 45 lessons throughout the academic year (during the first term in 2007). The School of Health Sciences provides IPE, general education, technical lectures, clinical training, and a graduation thesis, among other subjects, which forms a comprehensive, well-balanced educational curriculum between specialized education and holistic medical approaches.

3.2 Schedule of Teamwork Training

Simulated interprofessional training for health is provided to third-year students according to the following schedule.

First term

1. Introductory guidance (two lessons over 2 weeks): distribution of the training guidelines (Fig. 2a); briefing of the program; and introduction of academic staff (Fig. 2b)
2. Promotion of a sense of unity among students in groups (one lesson): selecting training facilities by students through a sports game (Fig. 3)

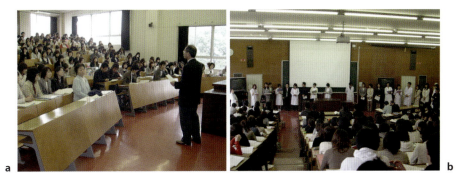

Fig. 2. **a** Overall guidance for a detailed explanation of the training program outline. **b** Introduction of academic staff for each group facilitator

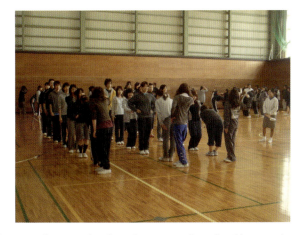

Fig. 3. Development of cooperation through sports, such as algorithm exercises

3. Overall guidance (two lessons over 2 weeks): introduction of training facilities and the allocation of students to the facilities based on the results of the game
4. Group work (ten lessons over 10 weeks): preparation of the training agenda and planning clinical training (and submission of this plan) (Fig. 4)

Latter term

5. Kick-off meeting and overall guidance prior to clinical training (one lesson): instructions on the clinical training program
6. Implementation of clinical training at above-assigned training facilities (2 days, equivalent to 10 lessons) (Fig. 5)

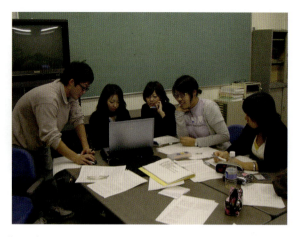

Fig. 4. Group discussions on medical or health care provided in the facility to develop a plan for clinical training

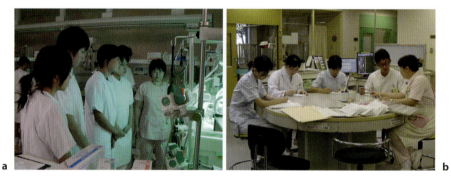

Fig. 5. Clinical training at a medical facility. Students are learning the practice of light treatment for a newborn (**a**) and have simulated team discussion with preceptor in the ward of a medical facility (**b**). Photos from "2007 Tokushoku GP Jireishu" (MEXT)

7. Group work (eight lessons over 8 weeks): preparation of a report on achievements and lessons learned from the clinical training program to be presented at the debriefing meeting (Fig. 6)
8. Debriefing meeting of the teamwork training (1 day, equivalent to five lessons): group presentations and general discussions (Fig. 7)
9. Group work (five lessons over 5 weeks): finalization of the clinical training reports to be compiled in a consolidated report
10. Wrap-up and general meeting (one lesson): submit the final report and conduct an evaluation survey

Interprofessional Education Initiatives at Gunma University

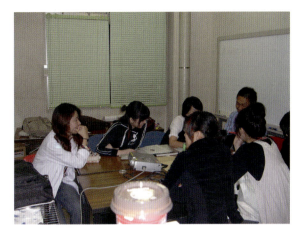

Fig. 6. Group learning where students and academic staff in charge of the group prepare for a debriefing meeting. Photo from "2007 Tokushoku GP Jireishu" (MEXT)

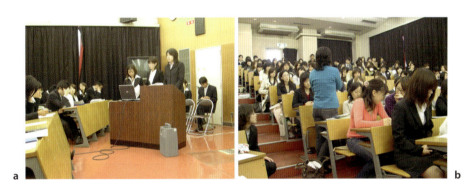

Fig. 7. Group presentations (**a**) and general discussions (**b**) at the debriefing meeting. Photos from "2007 Tokushoku GP Jireishu" (MEXT)

3.3 Facilities Where Clinical Training Is Provided (Wide Selection of Facilities to Address Issues in Modern Medicine and Welfare Services)

Modern medicine is provided by a variety of facilities ranging from university hospitals of advanced health care services to community/elderly care centers serving an aging society. In recent years, medical teams vary as well from the "top-down style" (e.g., emergency medical teams led by physicians) to "interprofessional" health care teams delivering community care services, including welfare and educational services. To encompass these situations, approximately 20 facilities are requested to cooperate with the clinical training; the facilities were selected based on the following seven fields: hospital medicine, community health care, care at home, rehabilitation, medical care for the mentally ill, pediatric care, and elderly care. These facilities have been playing a major role in delivering diversified health care services, and graduates from the School are working as key staff there. The facilities praise the School for producing competent health care professionals, and thus they are always ready to cooperate with the program, creating a desirable relationship.

4 Organization of the Program

4.1 Management of the Program

A total of six persons—two professors of the School of Health Sciences, who lead the project, and four associate professors (one from each department)—plan and manage the Teamwork Training Program. This management organization, Interprofessional Education Committee of Gunma University (IPEC-GU), as a driving force, contacts the selected training facilities, prepares an annual plan, organizes preparatory and management meetings, supervises academic staff who implement training with students, establishes standards for evaluation, conducts and analyzes the post-training evaluation surveys, and compiles reports on training. Roughly 20–30 academic staff members selected from the four departments implement the training of students according to the educational guidelines (Fig. 8).

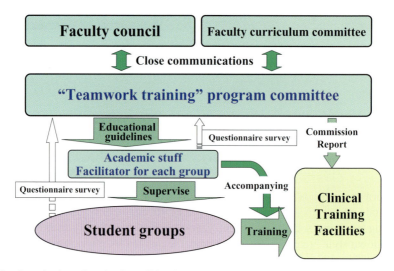

Fig. 8. Organization of academic staff for the IPE program

4.2 Participation of Students

A training group consists of eight students: four from the department of Nursing, two from Laboratory Sciences, and one each from Physical Therapy and Occupational Therapy—proportional to the enrollment capacity of each department. One academic staff member is assigned to each group. As all members of a group meet only once a week for this training, with the exception of the clinical training session at facilities, students and academic staff use a mailing list for close communication and coordination.

4.3 Support System in the School

During the 2 days of clinical training, at a kickoff discussion, and at a debriefing meeting, all regular classes in the School of Health Sciences are canceled, and its entire academic staff participates in the discussions and meetings. Achievements of the training program and the level of fulfillment of the educational agenda are reported once every 2 years at the annual Health Educational Workshop as part of faculty development in the School.

4.4 Efforts to Share the Importance and Values of the Program in the School of Health Sciences

4.4.1 Full Participation in General Discussions by All Departments

For the Teamwork Training Program, three general meetings are held: at the time of the first lesson, prior to clinical training, and for debriefing, with all departments participating in the discussions. At the debriefing meeting, reports of all training groups are presented and shared by all students, enabling the students to share the achievements of the program and the experiences of other groups in addition to their own.

4.4.2 Group Work Learning

During the group-work learning process, each group of students develops a clinical training plan closely supported by the academic staff member as facilitator. This arrangement enhances the quality of the plan. Each group takes advantage of the profiles of group members and develops a variety of educational approaches to interprofessional work.

4.4.3 Interaction Among Students and Academic Staff

A group consists of eight students from the four departments and one responsible academic staff. Students and academic staff interact with each other across departments. For instance, an academic member from the department of Laboratory Sciences teaches students from the department of Nursing. Close interaction among academic staff across departments (educational effect 3) is also achieved, and the values of the program are shared widely in the School of Health Sciences.

5 Characteristics of the Program

5.1 Efforts to Optimize the Training for Developing Students' Social Skills

5.1.1 Learning the Importance of Teamwork

Students learn the spirit of interprofessional work (educational goal 1) through fulfilling their roles in the team and working well together. Each group makes a presentation of its experiences at a debriefing meeting, which enables students to share experiences with each other. Students are expected to learn the importance of teamwork and improve their social skills throughout the program.

5.1.2 Enhancing the Effectiveness of the Clinical Training

A variety of practice sites are selected for the clinical training with a view to achieving educational goal 2 (practicing interprofessional work). In addition, simulated interprofessional training based on case scenarios is developed to optimize the short clinical training period.

5.1.3 Promoting Trust and Cooperation in a Team

Student groups compete with each other in a game held at the beginning of the training program. Groups with higher marks are given priority when selecting a health care facility for clinical training. Through this game, interaction among students across departments (educational effect 1) is achieved, leading to trust and cooperation among them.

5.1.4 Developing Presentation and Communication Skills

Students make presentations in front of a large number of people at a debriefing meeting after the clinical training. Students are expected to develop their presentation and communication skills through this experience.

5.1.5 Promoting Politeness and Appreciation

The level of achievement during the 2-day clinical training—the central part of the program—is determined by the quality and amount of preliminary work. Therefore, students are encouraged to make a site visit prior to the clinical training. They contact facility staff by themselves, arrange their visit, and hold a preliminary discussion with facility staff. After the clinical training, they send a report with a letter of appreciation to the facility. This helps promote professionalism, leading to the awareness of social responsibility (educational effect 2).

5.2 Response to Issues in Modern Medicine

It is important for all educational institutions of health professions to overcome adverse effects of the fragmentation of specialization. Because the turnover rates among young people are rapidly increasing and their professionalism is decreasing, it has been pointed out that career education should be designed in a way to reverse this trend. Students are expected to learn through clinical training the existence of a wide range of workplaces and diversified working modalities. The program contributes to the promotion of career education, an important agenda in modern medicine.

5.3 System Replicability as a Program Model and Educational Efforts for Continuity

Although this program requires the involvement of a large number of academic staff, it requires no specific equipment. Any educational institution can commence IPE if there are motivated academic staff, committed management, and good internal collaboration. It is possible for the School of Health Sciences to form interprofessional teams by itself because it contains four departments. However, it is also possible to organize teams across multiple universities and faculties and establish another model for IPE. Taking into account its advanced experience, Gunma University coordinates an IPE network and exchanges information with the Japan Interprofessional Working and Education Network (JIPWEN).

6 Efficacy of the Program

6.1 Assessment Mechanism of Educational Effects

To assess the effect of the training program objectively, an anonymous survey is conducted at the end of the training, asking students to evaluate the program and make comments. The results are shown in the following subsections.

6.1.1 Assessment of the Facilities Where Clinical Training Was Provided

The surveys that assessed the clinical training facilities in previous years indicated that more than 90% of students appreciated the experience and knowledge they obtained at the facilities. This suggested that there were well-developed educational capacities at these facilities.

6.1.2 Assessment of Achievement Levels

The survey to assess achievement levels contained 10 questions on self-assessment (Table 1) of the students' educational achievements. Students rated each question on a four-point scale of understanding: 4, "I fully understood"; 3, "I understood"; 2, "I did not understand well"; 1, "I did not understand at all." Thus, there were two positive and two negative responses. Figure 9 shows the results obtained in 2007. The same tendency has been observed across years. More than 90% of respondents "fully understood" or "understood" the importance of teamwork (Fig. 9A). This indicated that educational goal I (the spirit of interprofessional work) was achieved and that students effectively met the educational goal of the program. In contrast, fewer than 50% of respondents "understood" their profession's role and uniqueness (Fig. 9B). One possible reason was that students might have mixed up the purposes of multiple subjects, including the expertise clinical training subject held independently by each department, that was ongoing in parallel with the IPE training. Negative responses decreased year by year after we emphasized the IPE purpose at the guidance sessions. At the same time, however, it was noted that its primary reason was the students' dissatisfaction with gaining the skills for interprofessional work. Thus, a fundamental improvement plan was developed (discussed below).

Table 1. Questions in the survey conducted after the training session[a]

1. Organization of the facility
2. Function of the facility
3. Roles of each profession in the facility
4. Operations and tasks of each profession in the facility
5. Collaboration among professionals working in the facility
6. Your profession's role and uniqueness
7. Teamwork experienced in the training facility
8. Membership and leadership in group activities
9. Teamwork required in various fields
10. Importance of teamwork

[a] Regarding the above questions, we asked students to assess their levels of understanding on a four-point scale, as described previously[6]

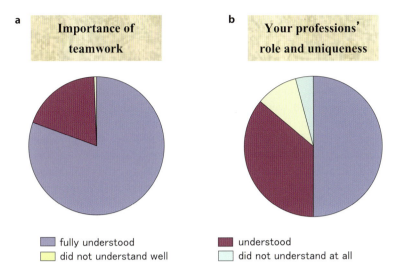

Fig. 9. Results of the assessment questionnaire conducted after the training session in 2007. More than 70% of students "fully understood" the "importance of teamwork" (question 10) (**a**), whereas fewer than 50% of respondents "fully understood" "*their* profession's role and uniqueness" (question 6) (**b**)

In the survey, students of the School of the Health Sciences repeatedly pointed out the need for medical students' participation in the IPE training. For instance, after the teamwork training in 2006, comments included the following: "It is necessary for the School of Medicine to work together with the School of Health Sciences—the departments of Nursing, Laboratory Sciences, Physical Therapy, and Occupational Therapy. Without medical students, it is difficult to learn the essence and reality of teamwork training." Medical students—who as physicians ultimately lead teamwork efforts—did not participate in the IPE training due to curriculum constraints of the School of Medicine.

Academic staff members in charge of training groups as facilitators were also asked their opinion regarding participation in group work and collaboration of facilities as well as their advice for improvement. Training groups assisted by motivated academic staff are likely to make excellent presentations. Uncommitted academic staff members often receive low marks or complaints from many students. Feedback with advice to each staff member was important to ensure the quality of the group's work. Academic staff members' opinions about training facilities were always taken into consideration when selecting practice sites for the next training session. The survey results confirmed that academic staff and students closely exchange opinions across departments, one of the achievements of the program (educational effect 3).

6.2 Plan for Further Development

6.2.1 Simulated Interprofessional Training Based on Case Scenarios

As mentioned above, students did not understand well their specific roles in interprofessional work and were dissatisfied with the Teamwork Training Program. Seemingly, they were unhappy by the lack of opportunities to treat patients as specialists. It was difficult to secure enough practice time for each student owing to the time constraint and the uncertainty of actual clinical settings. To overcome this deficit, it has been decided to introduce a modality called "simulated interprofessional training based on case scenarios." The teamwork training here replicates it into the group work training to achieve educational goal 2, gaining the skills for interprofessional work. Case scenarios common at facilities are developed in advance, and students are expected to deliberate and play their roles in the simulation.

6.2.2 Joint Training with Students from the School of Medicine

It was difficult for students of the School of Medicine to participate throughout the group work sessions because of their medical curriculum. As a first step to promote medical students' participation, it was proposed that some elements of the teamwork training be designated as elective subjects for second-year medical students. Elements include the simulated interprofessional training based on care scenarios, the clinical training, and the debriefing meeting where medical students join the group of students from the School of Health Science. First-year medical students are given information on IPE (elective subject for medical students), and second-year medical students can choose to register if they are interested.

6.2.3 Networking for Interprofessional Education with Medical Facilities and Other Universities

- *Networking with facilities for information exchange and consultation through organizing joint conferences.* Debriefing meetings, where training achievements are shared and information is exchanged among groups, have been held only in the School of Health Sciences. However, it is crucial to adapt the training to rapidly progressing/changing medical practice on the ground. Therefore, joint conferences are proposed with the preceptor staff of training-supporting facilities.
- *IPE networking with other universities.* This program is not large in scale but is expected to bring about considerable educational effects. Most educational

institutions could introduce a similar program without modifying their curricula substantially. To publicize the program as an advanced model, the School has planned to develop a website, improve curriculum guidelines, and publish educational materials. It has also planned to organize seminars by inviting lecturers who are involved in similar programs, such as "Community-based Interprofessional Training" (Sapporo Medical University), "Educational Initiative to Facilitate the Integration of Health, Medicine, and Welfare" (Saitama Prefectural University), and "Education for Multiple Health Care Professionals" (Jikei University School of Medicine). These seminars will help develop an extensive network of interprofessional education. With this initiative, the JIPWEN was established in June 2008.

7 Discussion

An increasing number of Japanese universities are incorporating interprofessional education into their curricula. Most Japanese universities provide it in the form of lectures. Even a short-term training program may have a positive effect on students' knowledge, interests, and attitudes.[1] Our School of Health Sciences has long had a clinical training program in which all students across departments have participated. The present program was constructed originally and implemented. Recently, IPE information has been obtained through the JIPWEN and other overseas networks, including the Centre for the Advancement of Interprofessional Education (CAIPE), European Interprofessional Education Network (EIPEN), Australasian Interprofessional Practice and Education Network (AIPPEN), and International Association for Interprofessional Education and Collaborative Practice (InterEd). This has allowed us to understand the remarkable progress in IPE and related research over the past decade.[3] To compare our IPE program with other training programs in and outside of Japan, it may be important to write articles about the Gunma IPE program, increasing visibility of the program. To assess the achievement levels of the programme we developed a questionnaire of 10 items, and we have recently shown that those were categorized into four subscales,[6] and suggested that the four subscales measure "understanding" well, and may take into account the development of interprofessional education programmes with clinical training in various facilities.[6]

The School of Health Sciences implemented the Teamwork Training Program, the core of IPE, in 1999. All of the program's details—including the training contents, modalities, materials, and assessment methods—were originally developed by the School. The activities were undertaken only locally, however, and its information was not publicized or shared widely. In 2007, the program was given a Good Practice (GP) award by the Ministry of Education, Culture, Sports, Science, and Technology (MEXT) and a grant-in-aid was provided. Hammnick et al. suggested, in a review, that funding enables evaluations of IPE to make a real contribution to its further development.[2] The educational research grants helped the School pay attention to what was taking place outside the university, to recognize the status of IPE in other universities, and to obtain information about international education and research programs and IPE networks among educational institutions inside and outside Japan. Thus, good financial support may indeed contribute to intensifying and expanding IPE activities.

The quality of IPE is influenced by the training modules.[3] In our IPE program, clinical training modules depend on facilities that support training. Most of the facilities have continuously accepted students, and hence those facilities qualified in the seven fields mentioned above have been consistently available for training over the 9 years of the program, with some minor changes. Each facility developed original modules of its own for training. Retaining an IPE rather than a topical content focus is essential.[3] To adapt the training to rapid progress and changes in clinical practice, it is important to organize joint conferences with facilities' preceptor staff and to provide consistent, effective practical training.

In the survey, students of the School of the Health Sciences repeatedly pointed out the need for medical students' participation in IPE training. Commitment to teamwork medicine and IPE is poor in the medical school.[4] There are many barriers to the engagement of doctors in collaborative processes including specific powers, status, professional socialization, and decision-making responsibility. It has been pointed out that it is critical for educators to deal with the doctor dilemma: how and why will doctors collaborate?[5] The Schools of Medicine and Health Sciences are located on the same campus of Gunma University, and there has been a long history of interaction in sports, music, and other extracurricular activities. Apparently, the School of Medicine was not reluctant to participate in the IPE program, but the difficulty of integrating the curricula of the two schools has prevented participation of medical students.[6]

The acquisition of Competitive Research Grants from MEXT has brought changes in the academic setting of the faculty of medicine, resulting in the development of a cooperative system among the academic staff in the faculty and in partial integration of the curricula. Accordingly, the first joint training program was implemented during the 2008 academic year. It was revealed that, in addition to providing financial support, public funding helped improve the IPE environment. To examine the significance of IPE for students in the School of Medicine, the School will follow those who have undergone the training program to assess their socialization as physicians.

Acknowledgments The authors are grateful to Professor Hirokazu Murakami, former Dean of the School of Health Science; Professor Kuniaki Takada, President of the University; and Professor Jun-ichi Tamura and Professor Noriyuki Koibuchi for their kind support of this program. We also thank Dr. Seiji Ozawa, former Vice President of Gunma University, for his kind help and assistance for this program. This work was supported in part by a grant, a Good Practice (GP) entitled "Interprofessional Education between Students Majoring in Health Sciences and Medicine Incorporating a Simulation Training Approach" from the Ministry of Education, Culture, Sports, Science, and Technology (MEXT).

References

1. Hoffman SJ, Harnish D (2007) The merit of mandatory interprofessional education for pre-health professional students. Med Teach 29:e235–e242
2. Hammick M, Freeth D, Koppel I, et al (2007) A best evidence systematic review of interprofessional education: BEME Guide no. 9. Med Teach 29:735–751
3. Johnston G, Banks S (2000) Interprofessional learning modules at Dalhousie University. J Health Adm Educ 18:407–427
4. Curran VR, Sharpe D, Forristall J (2007) Attitudes of health sciences faculty members towards interprofessional teamwork and education. Med Educ 41:892–896
5. Whitehead C (2007) The doctor dilemma in interprofessional education and care: how and why will physicians collaborate? Med Educ 41:1010–1016
6. Ogawara H, Hayashi, T, Asakawa Y, et al (2009) Systematic inclusion of mandatory interprofessional education in health professions curricula at Gunma University: a report of student self-assessment in a nine-year implementation. Hum Resour Health 7:60

Annex 1. Comparison among IPE[a] initiatives inplemented in the JIPWEN Universities

	Sapporo Medical University	Niigata University of Health and Welfare	University of Tsukuba	Saitama Prefectural University	Tokyo Jikeikai Medical University
Title	Team-based practical training program	Integrated general seminar	Experience-based educational program	Community-based interprofessional education	The nursing care practice for medical studer.
Backgrounds (common)					
Advanced and specialized medical technology				+	
Decrease in birth rate			+	+	
Aging population	+	+	+	+	
Lifestyle-related illnesses	+		+	+	
Diversity and complexity of illness	+		+	+	
Higher demands for a better quality of medical care	+	+	+	+	
Requirement for welfare service		+	+	+	
Child abuse				+	
Accidents					
Quality down due to increase in number of some health professions					
Backgrounds (specific)	Uneven distribution of medical personnels	Excellencent QOL supporters' training	Diversification of patients' need	Establishment through incorporation with UK CAIPE[b]	Mr. Takaki, the establishing person of the university, expanded the British patient-centere medicine
Objectives or goals	Commnity health care	Close collaboration among medical and welfare professionals	Close cooperation among health care professions to provide comprehensive and composite health services	High-quality health and social care professionals who understand the need for working in cooperation with professionals in other disciplines and are competent in working with them	Do not see the disease; see the patient

[a] IPE: Interprofessional education; the term "IPE" is introduced to Japan in 1996, [b] Centre for the Advancement of Interprofessional Education
[c] Professionals of welfare include social welfare

Keio University	Chiba University	Kitasato University	Kobe University	Gunma University
The promotion program for training high quality medical professionals	Educationan program for training autonomous healthcare professionals	The interprofessional team-based medical education program	Becoming interprofessional	Simulated interprofessional training among students of different professions in health sciences
		+	+	+
			+	
		+	+	+
		+	+	
			+	
	+	+	+	+
		+	+	+
			+	
			+	
years are required for pharmaceutical studnents (2006) high quality of ethics and humanity capability of solving problems	Independent education systems pursued highly specialized felds of study among 3 departments	Students of 14 different types of health-related professions are learning.	* natural disasters * WHO stressed the importance of "learning together" in 1987 * demand for cost-effective, patient-cetered, safe and reliable, high quality services across institutional and community health care	Holistic medical approaches
presentation skill information technology	patient (user)-centered medicine, fostering of communication skills, ethical sensitivity, and problem-solving skills	1) understanding the knowledge, skills, and expertise of other professions 2) acquiring the capacity to liaise and collaborate with other professions 3) acquiring the capacity to serve patients holistically	1) understand the term "interprofessional" 2) understand and respect the roles of different health professions 3) skill-mix 4) understand meanings and values of collaboration, develop a positive attitude towards it 5) develop collaborative skills (i.e. in clinical practice) 6) IPW perspective in the light of reforms and changes in health and welfare	Expriencing being a part of a health care team Leaning the inteprofessional work in clinical practice

Annex 1. (continued)

	Sapporo Medical University	Niigata University of Health and Welfare	University of Tsukuba	Saitama Prefectural University	Tokyo Jikeikai Medical University
Starting year	2004	2004	2004	1999	1989
Majors of participating students		75 (2008)			
Medicine (number of students)	+		+ (100): 3rd year		+
Nursing	+		+ (80): 4th year	+	+
Laboratory Sciences			+ (40): 4th year	+	
Physical Therapy	+	+		+	
Occupational Therapy	+	+		+	
Speech therapy		+			
Pharmacy					
Nutrition		+			
Social work (case-work)				+	
Professionals of welfare[c]		+		+	
Oral health				+	
Nurture				+	
Committee driving IPE mainly	Medicine and health professionals	Health and welfare professionals	Medicine	SPU faculty member	The educational committee
Main IPE style	Practice training	Lectures	Practice training	Practice training	Practice
Years involved	1 year	4 years	5 years for medicine	2 years (1st and 4th)	5 years for medicine 4 for nursing
Curricular activitiy	Extracurricular	Intracurricular	Intracurricular	Intracurricular	Intracurricular
Contents (duration/ months)	Practice trainiing in the rural areas	Lecture form trainig subject	Program to develop IP competence	Interprofessional courses (one of 4 coursed described below)	Reflective practice: the way of observing norms, reflecting on yourself, and improving your behavior
	Sequential program within a year * preparatry training period (6): team construction * residential community internship program (4) * community health care seminors	Sequential program in all years * 1st year: basic seminor (lecture) * 2nd and 3rd years: subjects related to IPE * 4th year: integrated generl seminor Twice a week for 7 weeks/group discussion	Sequential program in 5 years * 1st year: early exposure * 2nd year: home medical care (tutorial) * 3rd year: case colloquium (teamwork) * 4th year: experiencing other health professionals * 5th year: community-based medicine clerkship	Human care course: 1st year students lectures and group discussion Field activities course: 1st year students practice training at various human care facilities outside of university IP work course: 4th year students clinical or social case discussion for 4 days at approximately 90 community facilities in Saitama Prefecture Also, the student should learn several courses of other profession	Sequential program in all years * 1st year: community seviceo for handicapped program * 2nd year: care for incurable case * 3rd year: health care at home * 4th year: working at a hospital * 5th year: workshop for patient safety For nursing students workshop is learnt at 4th year

...eio University	Chiba University	Kitasato University	Kobe University	Gunma University
)06	2007	2006	2002	1997
)0–118 students for each seminor (2008)		14 different health-related professions 1,000 students for lecture 1,200 students for drill		
(8–20)	+	+	+ (100) for only 4th year	+ (30)
(28–50)	+	+	+ (80)	+ (80)
		+	+ (40)	+ (40)
		+	+ (20)	+ (20)
		+	+ (20)	+ (20)
		+		
(30–41)	+	+	+	
		+		
		+		
		+		
GL Committee	The Interprofessional Education Promotion Committee	2 committees under vice president, leader * Team-based medicine education committee (8 members) * Implementation committee of team-based medical exercise (42 members)	Kobe University Interprofessional Education for Collaborative Work Center (KIPEC)	Interprofessional Education Committee of Gunma University (IPEC-GU)
...eminors (lecture and group works)	Lectures, drills, and practical training	Drill and lectures	Lecture and exercise training	Lecture and pratice training
...year for whole students	4 years	2 years (1st and 3rd or 4th)	4 years	2 years (1st and 3rd)
...xtracurricular	Intracurricular	Intracurricular lectures & extracurricular drill	Intra- and extracurricular	Intracurricular
...seminors (2008)	Multi-stage, long-term, systemic program	Collaboration among 14 different health-related professions	Learn together to work together	Simulated interprofessional training
...day for each seminors	Step 1 Sharing: communication skill Step 2 Creation: team building & collaboration Step 3 Solution: decision making Step 4 Integration: patients center practice	Introduction to team-based medicine: real-time two-way-dialogue-style online lectures for 1st year students All Kitasato team-based medical drill (2 days): drill exercise for 3rd or 4th year students	Sequential program in all years (intracurricular) * 1st year: lecture, trainig and early exposure(1) * 2nd year: lecture for international and disaster * 3rd year: IPW-exercise * 4th year: clinical-based IPW training Extracurricular activities IPW week IPW day	*1st year: lectures *3rd year: practice training
	step by step progression			

133

Annex 1. (continued)

	Sapporo Medical University	Niigata University of Health and Welfare	University of Tsukuba	Saitama Prefectural University	Tokyo Jikeikai Medical Universi
Institutions supporting IPE outside	* medicla facility * prefectural government * local administration offices * local residents * community circls	* medicla assiciation (web discussion) * prefectural government		In field activities course * hospital * social welfare institution * community care center * voluntary association * local government	nurse stations
Evaluation				IP work course	
Objectives or items	* Achievements of understanding * Attitudes for IPW	* Achievements of understanding * Attitudes for IPW	* Achievements of understanding * Attitudes for IPW	* Achievements of understanding (learning) * Attitudes for IPW (behavior)	* Evaluation of the program
Methods	* VAS * Comparison between before and after	Scoring	Scoring	* Scoring * Comparison between before and after the IP work course	* Scoring
Outcome	Significant effects	Significant effects	Significant effects	Significant effects	Over one third of students evaluated goo
Others	* IPE programs delivered separately Medicine: 1st year, class work 5–6th year, resident communitiy health care training Health sciences: team-based practical training			Four subject groups liberal arts courses department basic courses department specialized courses interprofessional subjects In addition, each student needs to take another department courses (two units)	

Keio University	Chiba University	Kitasato University	Kobe University	Gunma University
	* Chiba University Hospital * Medical institutions out side * Patient's self-help groups * Social and welfare institutions * Home visit nursing stations * Pharmacies * Public health centers	4 university-affiliated hospitals	Kobe Pharmaceutical University	20 facilities out side of University Hospital medicine, community health care, care at home, rehabilitation, medical care for the mentally ill, pediatric care, elderly care
* Achievements of understanding * Attitudes for IPW	* Achievements of understanding * Attitudes for IPW	* Achievements of understanding	Attitudes for IPW	Achievements of understanding
Scoring	Report and group interview Scoring	Scoring	Scoring (RIPLS)	Scoring
	Significant effects	Every score showed over 3 points out of 4	Significant effects	Significant effects
Students from multiple universities attend on the registration		"Team-based clinical training" will be inplemented in four university-affiliated hospitals		

Subject Index

a
achievement level   124
actual patient   48
adult-learning theories   109
All-Kitasato Team-Based Medical Drill   76, 80, 81, 88, 89
anticancer drug overdose   59
assessment of the program   89
attitude toward collaboration   102
Australasian Interprofessional Practice and Education Network (AIPPEN)   127

b
Basic Seminar I   15
Basic Seminar II   15
better-quality medical care   4
bioethics   58
Board of Directors   88
British-type patient-centered medicine   50

c
CAIPE   127
care colloquium (teamwork training course)   29, 31
career development   3
Case scenario   126
Center of Planning and Coordination for Medical Education (PCME)   35
Centre for the Advancement of Interprofessional Education (CAIPE)   41
cerebrovascular medicine   82
chemotherapy outpatient care at home   92
Child Rearing in the Community   53
clinical case   44
clinical clerkship   26
clinical engineering technologist   77
clinical laboratory technician   77

clinical training center for the whole university   92
collaboration   98
collaboration among health professionals   99
collaborative capability   53
collaborative capacities   110
collaborative competencies   99
collaborative medicine   77
collaborative practice   95
collaborative teamwork   101
Committee of School Heads   88
Committee on Interprofessional Education of the School of Medicine and Medical Sciences   35
communicating   47
communication skills   65, 67, 70
communication theory   84, 86
communication training   27, 28
community   41, 51
community health and welfare institution visit   27, 28
community health care   1
community resident   16
community-based medicine clerkship   29, 32
conference   41
consortium   59
cooperation   45
cooperation among organizations   99
cooperation skill   20
critical path   92
curriculum   97
curriculum development   6

d
decision-making process   88
diabetes   19
diabetes mellitus (DM) medical management   82
disaster medicine   82

e

early exposure   27, 28
educational goal   15
educational philosophy   72
educational workshop   54
elective (semi-mandatory) course   89
emergency medicine   82
epidemiological and demographic profiles   93
essentials for medical professionals   26
essentials for Medical Professionals course   28
ethical sensitivity   65, 67, 70
ethics   58
European Interprofessional Education Network (EIPEN)   127
evaluation   43
evaluation process   71
examples of team-based medicine, medical ethics, medical safety   84
experience of other medical profession's work   29
experience-based educational program   22
experience-based learning   108
experiencing old age   27
experiencing old age, pregnancy   28
experiencing other health professionals' work   31
extracurricular activities   108

f

facilitation technique   110
facilitators   58, 82, 87
facilitator training seminars   42
faculty development (FD)   35
Faculty of Health Sciences   102
feedback   55
feedback lecture   60
Field Activities course   42
future professions   18

g

general instructional objective (GIO)   79
geriatric medicine   82
Good Practice (GP) award   127
group work   47, 117, 118
Gunma University   113

h

14 health-related professions   77
handicapped   52

handicapped children   52
Health Administration Office   41
health and social care professional   40
Health and Sports   14
health and welfare system   86
health care at home   52
health care practice   4
health care system   84
health education   8
Health Educational Workshop   121
Health Professions Education and Research Coordination Committee (HPERCC)   91
health promotion   8
health supervisor   77
hidden curriculum   51
holistic manner   8
holistic medicine   113
holistically   44
home care   59
home medical care course   29, 30
Hospital Clinical Training Center   93
hospital ward visit   27, 28
Human Care course   41
humanity   58
hypertension   19

i

Implementation Committee of Team-Based Medical Exercise   87
importance of teamwork   124
incurable patient   52
infection control   82, 92
information and communication technologies (ICT)   19
in-house clinical education center   92
inpatient experience   27, 28
Integrated General Seminar   13, 17, 18
integrated service   41
international and disaster health care   103, 106
international and disaster health care activities   103
International Association for Interprofessional Education and Collaborative Practice (InterEd)   101
international in disaster health care   96
interprofessional clinical practice   96
interprofessional competence   22, 26
interprofessional competencies   110
interprofessional course   41
interprofessional education (IPE)   1, 13, 15, 58, 115

Subject Index

Interprofessional Education Committee of Gunma University (IPEC-GU) 120
Interprofessional Education Promotion Committee 70
interprofessional education/learning (IPE/L) 95
interprofessional team 96
Interprofessional Team-Based Medical Education Program 76
interprofessional work (IPW) 26, 41, 98, 113
interprofessional work unit 28
interprofessional work units 27
interprofessionalism 73, 97
intraprofessional practice 44
Introduction to Team-Based Medicine 80, 84
Introduction to Team-Based Medicine lecture 76
IPE/L curriculum 99
IPW Club at Kobe University 108
IPW competencies 103
IPW Day 108
IPW education 97
IPW Week 108

j

Japan Association for Interprofessional Education (JAIPE) 20, 41, 103, 108
Japan Interprofessional Working and Education Network (JIPWEN) 103, 108, 123, 127
Jikei University School of Medicine 49, 50
joint curriculum 4
joint learning 99
joint seminar 58

k

Kinki Journal of Interprofessional Care 108
Kinki Team Treatment Forum 108
Kobe University Interprofessional Education for Collaborative Work Center (KIPEC) 103
Kitasato Institute 76
KJ method 82
Kobe Pharmaceutical University 102
Kobe University 95

l

lateral education 81
learning effects 46, 48
learning together 96
lecture 84
lifestyle-related disease 19
lifestyle-related disease management 82
lifestyle-related illness 4
local community staff 7
long-term nursing care 3

m

3P model 110
mandatory course 89
medical ethics 86
medical safety 86
medical student 125, 126
midwife 77
modern medicine 123
multidisciplinary care 16
multidisciplinary workplace 50
multiple departments 42

n

networking for interprofessional education 126
neurological incurable disease management 82
nurse 77
Nutrition Support Team 59
nutritional support 92

o

occupational therapist 77
Onomichi Medical Association 17
Oriental Medicine Research Center 92
orthoptist 77
other departments 18
other professions 45
outpatient escort program 27, 28
overall guidance 117
own profession 45

p

palliative care 59, 92
panel discussion 60
participation 45
partnership capacity 4
patient (user)-centered care 65
patient safety 52

patient safety workshop 55
patient-centered medical services 89
patient-centered medicine 66, 67, 77
patient-centered services 98
patient-centered, health service 77
patient–doctor relationship 26
patient-oriented and patient-centered approaches 48
pediatric oncology 82
pharmacist 77
physical therapist 77
physician 77
postplacement effects 43
practical learning 22
practical training 65, 70
practical training program 5
pre-event briefing for the facilitators 88
pregnancy 27
pre-on-the-job-training 20
preplacement effects 43
presage–process–product 110
presentation 60
presentation and communication skills 122
preventive medicine 8
problem-based learning (PBL) tutorial 26
problem-solving skills 65, 67, 70
profession's role and uniqueness 124
professional identity 78
professional roles 48
professionalism 26, 46
professions' cultures 50
professions' roles 46
Prosthetics & Orthotics and Assistive Technology 14
public health 3
public nurse 77

q
QOL supporter 14
quadriplegia 17
questionnaire results 61
questionnaire survey 18, 82

r
radiology technologist 77
real-time, two-way, dialogue-style, online lecture 76, 86
reflection 105
reflective learning 109
reflective practice 52
registered dietitian 77
residential community internship program 1

RIPLS 106
roles of a doctor 46

s
SBO achievement 90
School of Allied Heath Sciences 77
School of Health and Social Services 40
School of Health Sciences 114
School of Medicine 77, 102
School of Nursing 77
School of Pharmacy 77
self-assessment 124
self-assessment questionnaire 11
self-learning program 6
Severely Handicapped Children 53
SGL method 58
Shibasaburou Kitasato 76
simulated interprofessional training 116
simulated patient 16
skills required for collaboration 102
Small Group Learning (SGL) Committee 58
social needs for holistic and humanized health care 93
specific behavioral objective (SBO) 79
speech-language-hearing therapist 77
Support Program for Contemporary Education Needs 41
support system 70
systematic IPE program 51
System-wide Kitasato University Clinical Training Center 93
system-wide university center 92
system-wide University Clinical Education Center 76

t
tailor-made and individualized treatment 93
tailor-made medicine; gene therapy; regenerative medicine 86
teaching assistant 70
teaching/learning methods for IPW and IPE/L 101
team 45, 46
team members' profession 84
team-based 5
Team-Based Clinical Training 91
Team-Based Clinical Training Program 92
Team-Based Medical Education Committee 87
Team-Based Medical Education Forum 88

Subject Index

team-based medicine   77
team-based medicine forum   83
team-based residential community health care
    internship   2
team-building skill   110
teamwork training   114
terminal care   59
The Oriental Medical Research Center   93
timetable   81

u
undergraduate curriculum   95
understanding   45
understanding and knowledge   18

understanding of patients   46
United Kingdom   20
University of Tsukuba   22

v
vertical education   80

w
Working Group of the HPERCC   91
workplace   52, 56
World Health Organization (WHO)
    Collaborating Center for Traditional
    Medicine   92

Printed in Japan